3|15

D0057052

DISCARD

# THE
# LOW-CARB
# FRAUD

## T. Colin Campbell, PhD

### with *HOWARD JACOBSON, PhD*

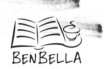

BenBella Books, Inc.
Dallas, Texas

BenBella

BenBella Books, Inc.
10300 N. Central Expressway
Suite #530
Dallas, TX 75231
www.benbellabooks.com

Send feedback to feedback@benbellabooks.com

Printed in the United States of America
10   9   8   7   6   5   4   3   2   1

**Library of Congress Cataloging-in-Publication Data**

Campbell, T. Colin, 1934–
   The low-carb fraud / T. Colin Campbell, PhD, with Howard Jacobson, PhD.
      pages cm
   Includes index.
   ISBN 978-1-940363-09-7 (trade cloth) — ISBN 978-1-940363-03-5 (electronic)
1. Low-carbohydrate diet. 2. Nutrition. 3. Prehistoric peoples—Food. I. Jacobson,
Howard, 1930–  II. Title.
   RM237.73.C36 2014
   613.2'833—dc23

                                                                    2013037793

Copyediting by Oriana Leckert
Proofreading by Chris Gage and Amy Zarkos
Indexing by Clive Pyne Book Indexing Services, Inc.
Cover image by Getty Images
Cover design by Bradford Foltz
Jacket design by Sarah Dombrowsky
Text design and composition by
Printed by Bang Printing

Distributed by Perseus Distribution
perseusdistribution.com

To place orders through Perseus Distribution:
Tel: 800-343-4499
Fax: 800-351-5073
E-mail: orderentry@perseusbooks.com

**Significant discounts for bulk sales are available. Please contact Glenn Yeffeth at glenn@benbellabooks.com or 214-750-3628.**

*To the promoters of the "low-carb" diet who*
*prompted me to write this book*

# CONTENTS

# THE LOW-CARB
# FRAUD

I t's no secret that Americans struggle with weight loss. Since 1980, when the rise in obesity first caught the attention of the media, the national rate of obesity has doubled.[1] Now, more than one-third of all U.S. adults are obese. And despite hundreds of new (or cleverly recycled) "solutions" hitting the shelves in book or prepackaged food form each year, we just can't seem to stem the tide. Our national weight problem is just the tip of the iceberg, however; being overweight is linked to some of the major causes of premature death, including heart disease, stroke, Type 2 diabetes, and some cancers.[2]

This book is primarily about low-carb diets—one of the more financially successful, and one of the most health-threatening, solutions proposed to meet our desire to shed pounds and become healthier. We'll discuss why the low-carb diet is so appealing, how we've been tricked in thinking it's healthy, and the truth about its health impacts. But this book is also concerned with the beliefs about nutrition that underlie those things: where the belief that carbs are bad came from, and why it has persisted despite so much evidence to the contrary.

There have almost always been fad diets with varying degrees of scientific merit, some more effective than others. Several decades ago, and still to a certain extent today, the most trusted advice was, essentially: eat less and exercise more. Weight loss was a matter of arithmetic—calorics in vs. calories out. But we were also told that dietary fat is the problem. Fat is what makes us, well, fat. So if we want to lose weight, all we have to do is consume less of it.

But as the national obesity rate rose, it was clear that this advice on fat just wasn't cutting it. The Standard American Diet (SAD) also wasn't cutting it. We needed to rethink the way we looked at proper nutrition. It was during the 1980s, in the wake of these rising concerns, that the low-carb movement began to take hold. It hit its stride in 1988, with the publication of Dr. Robert Atkins' *New Diet Revolution*, which was "new" only in that it followed Atkins' 1972 book, *Dr. Atkins' Diet Revolution*, which had not been especially successful in the marketplace. And this "new" book's contents represented an appealing alternate belief system about weight, nutrition, and health.

In a nutshell, the low-carb movement told adherents to severely limit their intake of carbohydrates and instead to get the lion's share of their calories from protein and fat. The problem with the SAD isn't fat, the book claims, but carbs—those found in bread, rice, and pasta, in fruit and starchy vegetables. The best way to lose weight, Atkins proclaims, is to cut back on carbs.

And it worked! By feasting on bacon and steak and butter, low-carb dieters actually did drop pounds. Which would be great, except for one important thing: the low-carb diet is not good for human health. Report after report has shown the ill effects of a high-protein, high-fat diet. It's just as bad, if not worse, than the SAD it seeks to replace.

In this book, I will explore a couple of important questions: Why do people think low-carb diets are a good idea? What's the truth behind the low-carb hype? What's the truly optimal diet for achieving an ideal weight while also obtaining health and longevity?

If there's one thing I hope you'll take away from this book, it's this: the low-carb diet's ability to bring about quick weight loss is far outweighed by the serious health problems that accompany such an animal foods–heavy diet.

## THE LOW-CARB APPEAL

I've spent more than forty years in experimental nutritional research, first at Virginia Tech and then at Cornell, keeping up with the latest discoveries and doing my own work, both in the lab and in the field. And as a nutritional researcher, I was surprised at first by the popularity and commercial success of the low-carb diet, especially given its serious flaws. The research on high-protein, high-fat diets has consistently demonstrated that they have disastrous health effects and fail to secure compliance and long-term weight loss. So I think it's useful to point out some factors that have contributed to these diets' appeal.

It's easy to imagine why dieters might be swayed—both then and now—by the idea of trying something radically different. Millions of Americans are on diets. Food manufacturers and marketers flood the marketplace with foods designed to help us lose weight and keep it off. Television features a steady stream of infomercials touting new gadgets, exercise routines, pills, and powders that can help us shed those unsightly pounds. And, apparently, none of it is working.

For a shocking visual, compare these two slides, taken from a CDC presentation. The first slide shows data from 1990 and is far from ideal:

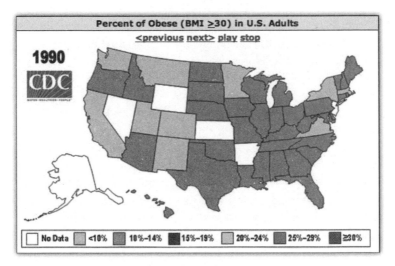

Forty-six of the fifty-two states and other U.S. jurisdictions report adult obesity rates between 10 and 20 percent, with obesity defined as a Body Mass Index (BMI) greater than 30. No state has an obesity rate above 20 percent.

Now look at the data from 2010:

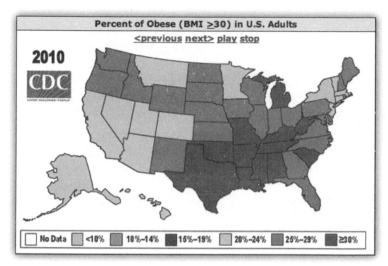

Just twenty years later, the thinnest states—with obesity rates under 25 percent—are all heavier than the heaviest states in 1990. And twelve states have cracked the 30-percent-plus mark.

The 2011 data, which haven't made it into the slideshow yet, include a new category: 35 percent or greater adult obesity rate. While it wasn't strictly necessary to add that category (Alabama came closest, with a 34.9 percent rate), the CDC were obviously planning ahead.[3]

Given the huge diet industry and its stunning lack of effectiveness, it's only natural that alternative approaches would gain popularity. Low-carb was the alternative that gained the largest amount of public acceptance and hence the greatest market share. But why did low-carb beat out the other nontraditional approaches?

One of the main answers is marketing rhetoric. On this point, I have to take my hat off to Robert Atkins. One of the major themes of my new book on nutritional science, *Whole: Rethinking the Science of Nutrition* (2013), is that paradigms, or entrenched ways of seeing the world, are devilishly hard to change. But Atkins and his supporters turned a century of nutritional wisdom on its head, framing dietary fat and cholesterol as nutritional heroes and attacking anyone who pointed to research showing otherwise. They gave Americans permission to eat huge amounts of some of the unhealthiest foods on the planet, and to do so not only without guilt, but with feelings of pride and superiority. The most impressive legacy of the Atkins craze is a linguistic achievement: coining the phrase "low-carb" and thereby turning most plant foods—which were previously considered the healthiest dietary choices—into dangerous and fattening no-nos.

The appeal of this was immediate, for obvious reasons. After decades of believing that losing weight was possible only by subsisting on salads, depressing lunches of grapefruit halves and fat-free cottage cheese, and diet sodas that taste like battery acid, people were told to eat as much as they wanted of their favorite foods: steak, bacon, butter, lard, cream cheese, olive oil, mayonnaise, and eggs. Eating was fun again!

And lo and behold, people found that—in the initial stages of this diet—they did lose weight. It seemed like the very foods that doctors and public officials had been warning against all those years actually promoted weight loss more effectively than the tasteless zero-fat processed foods that took all the joy from eating.

Not only could the Atkins followers sate their fat- and protein-cravings without guilt, they could even feel superior to the poor fools who were still eating salads, going to weight-loss meetings, and counting calories.

The Atkins Diet didn't just appeal to dieters; it was a boon to the meat, dairy, and egg industries as well. Not only could these companies now fend off public criticism of their products with low-carb "science," but they also saw greater sales.

# THE LOW-CARB LANDSCAPE

Not all low-carb diets are created equal, of course. The low-carb universe Atkins brought into being has grown to encompass many different diets and eating philosophies. But these are distinguished more by marketing than by substance—they all share the same fear and loathing of carbohydrates and recommend getting most of one's calories from protein and fat.

## *Atkins*

While Robert Atkins is the father of the modern low-carb movement, he didn't come up with the low-carb concept, something he freely admits in his books. The first person on record as having used this type of diet was William Banting, a British undertaker, in the 1860s. Banting, at the age of sixty-six, tried a low-carb diet at the recommendation of his physician, Dr. William Harvey. He lost body weight in the first few weeks and commented that he might like to continue the diet—though the longer-term results of Banting's alteration in diet, to my knowledge, were never clear. A few other medical practitioners experimented with low-carb diets with their patients over the next century, but the idea didn't enter mass public consciousness until the 1972 publication of *Dr. Atkins' Diet Revolution*.

Riding the wave of the low-carb diet's near-term success, Atkins authored many additional books before his passing in 2003. His professional career morphed into an empire; as of this writing in 2013, the 1988 *Dr. Atkins' New Diet Revolution* has sold more than 15 million copies, and Atkins Nutritionals, Inc., which produces and licenses Atkins-approved products, achieves annual sales in the millions of dollars. The Atkins Foundation funds research on the low-carb diet as it relates to obesity, Alzheimer's, prostate cancer, and other diseases. And the Atkins empire perseveres, despite its founder's death and a descent into bankruptcy following company mismanagement in 2004–2005; its present-day business still claims a big piece of the weight-loss market.

## Low-Carb Spinoffs

Smelling profits, many other doctors and authors put their own spin on the low-carb phenomenon and created their own books, diets, and products. Most prominent among them are Mary Dan and Michael Eades' *Protein Power* (1995), Barry Sears' *Enter the Zone* (1995), Peter D'Adamo's *Eat Right 4 Your Type* (1997), Loren Cordain's *The Paleo Diet* (2002), Arthur Agatson's *South Beach Diet* (2005), and Eric Westman's *The New Atkins for a New You* (2010). Like younger siblings struggling to stand out, these various authors and their supporters go to great lengths to distinguish their "correct" diet from the others. The *South Beach Diet* prefers olive oil to butter and emphasizes leaner cuts of meat. *Protein Power* adds lots of water and nutritional supplementation to compensate for the low-carb diet's inadequacies. *Enter the Zone* seemingly dismisses the low-carb idea by recommending "only" 30 percent protein but still relegates carbs to less than half your total calories. (That's still low carb!) Even *The Paleo Diet*, despite its positive emphasis on whole foods, is just another version of the same low-carb, high-protein, high-fat idea (see Appendix). These spinoffs all occupy the same very thin slice of the human diet continuum.

In addition to their carbophobia, these authors have two other things in common: no experience in scientific research and a vast fortune generated by the sales of their shakes, powders, extracts, oils, bars, and even chocolates, along with a second fortune amassed through licensing their trademarked seal of approval.

The net effect of all this differentiation and marketing has been the normalization of low carb on a cultural level. Restaurants routinely offer low-carb menu options. It's expected that someone watching their weight will bypass the dinner rolls. And whereas twenty years ago you would have raised an eyebrow (and a few concerns for your sanity) were you to sit down to a meal of bacon, butter, and beef for the purpose of shedding pounds, these days that's a perfectly normal approach to weight loss. When absurdities get repeated often enough, they start sounding like truth.

## THE REAL TRUTH ABOUT LOW-CARB DIETS

As I mentioned, low-carb diets are often pretty good at bringing about short-term weight loss. But that benefit comes with huge downsides. Low-carb diets target excess weight without paying attention to the underlying cause or causes of that weight, which leads to other symptoms. Low-carb diets often make those other symptoms, as well as the cause itself, worse.

What's the difference between attending to a cause and treating a symptom?

A brown lawn, for example, is a symptom. It's an unsightly, possibly embarrassing symptom that could get your neighbors shaking their heads and talking about you behind your back. "Look how he lets his lawn go," they might mutter. "Why doesn't he do something about it?"

So along comes the lawn-care specialist with a solution to your problem: green paint.

Voilà—problem solved!

Well, not exactly.

After painting the grass, your lawn will look green temporarily, but eventually the paint will wear or wash away, and then you have to call the lawn painter back in. The paint doesn't do anything about the poor health of the grass that led to it turning brown in the first place. And if the paint is toxic, it can even make the health of the grass worse. If you really want a lush green lawn—a *healthy* lawn that is *naturally* green—you need to improve the soil: add nutrients, remove toxins, water appropriately, and use the right grass seed for your environment. In other words, focus on the root causes, not just the visible symptoms.

If you want to lose weight, focusing solely on weight loss— as the low-carb diet does—is as unproductive as painting your lawn green.

The low-carb diet's first major flaw is that it's short term. Over the long term, low-carb diets don't fulfill their promise to dieters, which is that the diet will help them reduce their weight and sustain the change. Observation studies of populations overwhelmingly show that high-protein, high-fat diets, which reflect the long-term consumption of animal-based and highly processed food products, are associated with more health problems, many of which are associated with obesity.[4]

Americans are getting heavier and sicker, despite all the modern advances in medical care and technology. We're making no significant inroads in reducing rates of cancer, heart disease, stroke, diabetes, and dozens of other diseases intimately connected with obesity. It's just that, unlike diabetes or high blood pressure, obesity is a more visible symbol of the problem.

In truth, the obesity epidemic and the health crisis are two sides of the same coin. You can't solve one without solving the other. That's as true on an individual basis as it is for society as a whole. Obesity is a symptom, just like hypertension, clogged arteries, angina, chronic shortness of breath, belly pain, dizziness, constipation, and hundreds of others. Yet we largely, and wrongly, treat obesity as if it's a separate thing—a separate disease.

While there's a lot of overlap between a healthy body weight and overall health, they aren't synonymous. You can lose a lot of weight by getting cancer, and you can keep it off by dying, but I don't recommend that approach! Charitably, we could say that low-carb advocates are using weight loss as a Trojan Horse to get people to improve their diets and overall health—although there's little evidence for this generous interpretation. As Atkins himself was both obese and quite ill from the known consequences of a high-protein, high-fat diet at the time of his death,[5] it's clear that this community isn't taking seriously the damning data on long-term health outcomes.

Two original research papers reveal more about the consequences of the Atkins Diet than any others because they were published by supporters of the Atkins Diet and were funded by the Atkins organization. In one paper,[6] users of the Atkins diet, when compared to control subjects of "low-fat" dieters (dieters who were getting "only" 30 percent of their calories from fat), suffered more constipation (68 vs. 35 percent), more headaches (60 vs. 40 percent), more halitosis (38 vs. 8 percent), more muscle cramps (35 vs. 7 percent), more diarrhea (23 vs. 7 percent), more general weakness (25 vs. 8 percent), and more rashes (13 vs. 0 percent)—even those Atkins diet users who were taking vitamin supplements. In the other paper,[7] similar prevalences were seen for the Atkins dieters for constipation (63 percent), headaches (53 percent), and halitosis (51 percent).

These Atkins Diet side effects are consistent, and the research is quite convincing. That is, when compared with the already poor Standard American Diet (SAD), which is high in fat and protein, the Atkins Diet, even higher in fat and protein, leads to far more negative health outcomes, even in the short term.

So why do dieters still believe the low-carb hype? It has a lot to do with how convincing the low-carb movement's arguments *sound*—even though those arguments are consistently contradicted by the science.

## GARY TAUBES AND LOW-CARB SLEIGHT OF HAND

The best lies contain a kernel of truth, and that's certainly the case with the work of journalist Gary Taubes, by far the most eloquent and influential present-day spokesperson for the low-carb movement. Taubes' two bestselling books, *Good Calories,*

*Bad Calories* (2007) and *Why We Get Fat* (2011), make the low-carb case in an entertaining and, to many, compelling fashion.

Taubes is not, of course, the only person who writes in support of the low-carb diet, but I've chosen to center my critique around Taubes' writings because they represent the most comprehensive and evidence-rich expression of the low-carb idea. Taubes' work also provides—inadvertently, no doubt—a survey of many of the errors, logical problems, and sleights of hand common to low-carb advocates. By pointing out Taubes' errors and exposing his faulty reasoning, I hope to show the failures and intellectual poverty of the entire low-carb movement.

The first and perhaps most damning problem is the misreading of history and of the supposed link between low-fat diets and obesity. Taubes tackles this history in *Good Calories, Bad Calories*, a book billed as required reading for those interested in the evidence supporting a low-carb diet. While Taubes' account is certainly comprehensive, his interpretation is, shall we say, creative.

## WHERE TAUBES GETS IT RIGHT

Taubes begins with a kernel of truth, rightly pointing out that the effectiveness of counting calories is a myth. He also gets right some of the important history of the narrative on diet and health of the past five decades. And in his technical arguments on the underlying biochemistry of obesity, he gets some of these details right as well. But considered in isolation and spun into a narrative about the evils of carbs, these partial truths end up misleading rather than informing.

Taubes correctly points out that many early researchers, in the way they crafted their studies and reported their findings, were confusing the three main hypotheses for the causes of obesity and related illnesses: excess calories, excess fat, and excess carbs. According to the first hypothesis—by far the most common—we gain weight because we ingest more calories than we burn. This is the hypothesis I mentioned earlier, which you still hear being invoked today as if it's the most obvious thing in the world: "eat less, exercise more." Simple arithmetic. To his credit, Taubes does a masterful job of debunking this dangerous oversimplification.

Taubes goes on to argue, correctly, that creating long-term health by controlling calorie consumption does not work—a very important observation little understood by professionals and nonprofessionals alike. Most people cannot maintain significantly lower calorie consumption for long periods of time, even though they may be able to do so for a short while. That is, "diets" don't work—not because our willpower isn't up to it but because of our biological inability to healthfully maintain the substantially lower calorie consumption required to significantly decrease disease formation.[8] In any case, Taubes says, generally it is not the amount of calories consumed that matters most but the way calories are metabolized and distributed throughout the body (something we'll discuss in more depth in a few pages). In fact, Taubes argues that increased calorie consumption is the effect, not the cause of obesity—that we gain weight for other reasons and then require more calories to sustain that weight. Something else is causing obesity, and it is doing so by determining how our ingested calories are metabolized and used.

I applaud Taubes' demolishing the calorie hypothesis. In fact, I have long said that we should be careful not to emphasize the "calories in; calories out" hypothesis or describe calories in precise quantities as if they are physical entities, like molecules, that have structure and form, because doing so only gives them added importance.

A calorie is only a measure of energy contained within a molecule, especially within the chemical bonds that bind atoms. Think of a pile of wood. We know that there is energy in that pile of wood, but we cannot see or feel it. When we put a match to the wood, however, we feel that energy escaping as the wood bursts into flames. The calorie contents of nutrients are also determined by measuring the heat nutrients release when burned. To calculate this, macronutrients (fat, protein, and carbohydrates, the nutrients that provide the vast majority of the weight of food) are burned in controlled conditions in a laboratory, and the heat emitted—the temperature change—is measured as calories. (I prefer to call this property "energy" but will stick with "calories" here because of the term's broad familiarity.)

The amount of calories needed to produce a noticeable change in body weight, up or down, is very small—a notion that also sidetracks our emphasis on calories. A difference of fifty calories can be difficult to distinguish in the context of a day's total food intake; it's equivalent to an average of less than a teaspoon of oil per day. Yet a difference of fifty calories retained by the body per day can theoretically cause a gain or loss of five to ten pounds of body weight per year.[9] The problem is that *consumption* of calories does not equal *retention* of calories; retention of calories is not something we can consciously control by counting. So, in this respect, Taubes is correct: calorie intake or expenditure, except in the extreme, does not matter as our findings in China confirm.[10]

## WHERE TAUBES GETS IT WRONG

Taubes parts company with the evidence when he gets into the identification of where "bad calories" come from. Taubes sees excess consumption of calorie-contributing carbohydrates (the second of the three competing theories mentioned previously) as the root of all dietary evil. In his view, the consumption of sugar (table sugar or sucrose) and other carbohydrates (i.e., refined carbohydrates, such as starch and fructose) is responsible for the obesity epidemic in the United States and much of the rest of the world. And he blames this spike in carbohydrate consumption on the government's promotion of the third competing theory: that calories from fat make us fat. In Taubes' view, the fear of fat engendered by government low-fat policies drove the American public straight into the arms of a high-carb diet because it encouraged the replacement of this fat with carbohydrates. In short, Taubes says that too many carbs is the problem, while the government (or his interpretation of it) says the problem is too much fat.

Taubes argues on historical and scientific grounds that excess fat consumption cannot account for the alarming rise in obesity during the past thirty years the way government pronouncements suggest. Most readers will be familiar with the widespread recommendation to use low-fat foods, as well as the multitudes of "low-fat" food products on the market. Taubes presents a seemingly plausible account of how scientists working in this field got it wrong, partly because they were not very imaginative and partly because they became entrenched in a worldview that discouraged professional challenge against the much-publicized low-fat-focused hypothesis lest they be ridiculed or even risk losing their professional standing. Fat, not carbohydrates, Taubes says, should be our primary source of energy. Fat is good, he says, and not something merely dumped into a body reservoir that eventually becomes adipose tissue.

Before going further, let's consider what a carbohydrate actually is, especially because Taubes rather arrogantly lambasts scientists for not knowing the properties of this nutrient. (In my experience, it's really journalists like Taubes, corporate marketing agents, and even some clinicians who are confused about carbohydrates' definition and meaning.)

## *The Diversity of Carbohydrates*

Carbohydrate is a nutrient found almost exclusively in plants. It is a collection of simple to very complex chemical molecules. Simple carbohydrates include monosaccharides (like glucose, fructose, galactose, mannose, etc.) and disaccharides, which are made up of two chemically bonded monosaccharides (like sucrose [table sugar, made from glucose and fructose] and lactose [milk sugar, made from glucose and galactose]). Linked chains, or polymers, of three or more monosaccharides are called polysaccharides. Glucose (the same molecule as in blood sugar) is the most common monosaccharide unit in polysaccharide chains, with fructose being nearly as common in some foods. Starch, which is the primary polysaccharide in foods like potatoes and cereal grains, is a network of long chains of glucose molecules.

Monosaccharides and disaccharides are often considered "simple" carbohydrates because their molecular size is small, they readily dissolve in water, and they are easily digested and absorbed into the bloodstream. Some people infer that starches are also "simple" because they, too, dissolve in water (though they turn it into a gel or paste) and are readily broken down during digestion into glucose, which is then absorbed into the bloodstream.

Other carbohydrate types are much more complex. Elaborate networks of polymers are formed from chains of monosaccharides, sometimes also including amino acid and fat-like molecular side chains. These polymer networks exhibit a wide variety of chemical, physical, and nutritional properties. A large group of substances generally referred to as the dietary fiber group, for example, are, unlike their simple carbohydrate cousins, generally not digested and absorbed in the gut. Nonetheless, these complex, fiber-like substances still participate in vitally important biological activities: they interact with intestinal microorganisms that break them down into products that benefit the rest of the body, especially the intestines. Indeed, simple and complex carbohydrates, when working together, provide diverse health benefits, including the provision of energy.

Whenever we encounter diversity in nature, we should be slow to dismiss it as unnecessary or unfortunate. A broad spectrum of carbohydrate digestibility and function is very important: it allows the body to adapt to different conditions, ranging from the need for a quick burst of energy to the facilitation of digestion and absorption of other nutrients in the gut.

It's true that sucrose, the simple disaccharide that comprises table sugar, can be harmful when consumed in isolation. Sucrose is known to have little or no useful health value when extracted from sugar cane and sugar beet plants and added in isolated form to other foods. High-fructose corn syrup is another simple monosaccharide of more recent commercial vintage and exploitation. The latest studies suggest that its effects are as bad as those of sucrose,[11] if not worse.[12]

In order to use this evidence in support of the low-carb movement, Taubes performs a bit of sleight of hand, the crux of which is: refined sugar is bad, therefore all foods that contain sugars (i.e., carbs) are bad. This is poor logic even in the classical sense. We can also highlight the flaws in this reasoning by considering another carbohydrate found in plant food—fiber—and comparing its health effects when in its natural state and when processed, isolated, and consumed as a substance separate from that natural state.

Dietary fiber is extracted from all kinds of whole plants in order to add it to muffins and other baked goods as "bran." Marketers then claim health benefits from these baked goods, citing the research evidence on the goodness of fiber. But bran doesn't help us when it's been extracted from whole plants and then stuck into processed and fragmented foods like breads and breakfast cereals. Although there is some evidence that bran supplements may reduce certain indicators of serious health problems, I find no evidence that, over the long term, this is a good option for actually preventing or treating these problems.[13]

*Whole* foods that contain dietary fiber, in its many complex forms, *are* associated with lower incidence of colon cancer, lower blood cholesterol, and lower breast cancer–inducing estrogen levels. The use of bran isolated from these foods is more about marketing than health. This holds true for many isolated nutrients, which either have no positive health benefits or actually result in damaging effects.

If Taubes and his low-carb compatriots are against ingesting *refined* (i.e., extracted) sugars, they should say so, and I'd be among the first to support their crusade to eliminate those sugars from our diets. But instead, they tar the entire class of carbohydrates with the same brush, which is an intellectually superficial and dishonest move. (Taubes is more careful than some other low-carb cheerleaders, but not completely so. He should be proactively emphasizing this discrepancy, not allowing it to smolder just below the public narrative.)

Because fruits, vegetables, and whole grains are all high in carbohydrates, lumping all carbs together as unhealthy means demonizing plant-based foods as well as simple sugars. A diet low in carbohydrates is unavoidably a diet high in fat, especially saturated fat, because eliminating carbohydrates means relying on large quantities of animal-based products for energy and other nutritional benefits. Virtually by definition, therefore, a low-carb diet emphasizes the consumption of animal-based foods, while a low-fat diet emphasizes the consumption of plant-based foods. In my experience, it is this emphasis given to animal-based foods in low-carb (and thus high-protein, high-fat) diets that is the chief motivation of low-carb advocates.

The dramatic shift in consumption suggested by Taubes' oversimplification of the definition and meaning of carbohydrates has momentous consequences. Not only does shifting to a diet low in carbs severely minimize our intake of antioxidants, complex carbohydrates, vitamins, and certain minerals, it also shifts our dietary source of energy from carbohydrates to fat and encourages consumption of protein far above the required amount.

Why is this such a terrible thing? Because the foods we choose to meet our energy needs make a big difference in whether we experience good or ill health.

## *Number of Calories Versus Source of Calories*

If by "good and bad calories," Taubes means "good and bad sources of energy"—in effect, good and bad foods—he and I agree, at least in principle. Plant- and animal-based foods are hugely different in terms of their nutrient contents, and watching what foods you consume is far more important than obsessing over calorie-counting without respect to where those calories come from.

Take, for example, our research into the effect of dietary protein on cancer growth in experimental animals, involving about twenty-five individual experiments conducted over about thirty years. The animals consuming the lowest amount of protein (5 percent of total calories) had far less cancer than their higher-protein-consuming counterparts, while consuming an average of 2 to 3 percent *more* total calories (or, as I prefer to say, more total energy). This is an important observation: more calories consumed, but less cancer.

It was not easy to convince some of my colleagues of this finding because of their long-standing and almost certain belief that our conclusion should have been exactly the opposite: that increased calories lead to increased rates of cancer (as well as other disease). These beliefs on the calorie-cancer connection were based on prior experimental studies, which showed reduced cancer occurrence when calorie consumption was reduced by a hefty 20 to 30 percent or more.[14]

Our finding that more calories could also mean less cancer was initially puzzling to us, too. The reason for this result, we learned through additional studies, was the effect of dietary protein on the body's distribution and use of the consumed energy. A low-protein diet (such as a whole food, plant-based diet) increases the proportion of dietary calories expended either as body heat[15] or through voluntary physical activity,[16] thus sparing the storage of this energy as body fat. Our low-protein experimental animals consumed more oxygen and formed more of a highly specialized tissue (known as *brown adipose tissue*), which diverts calories/energy away from the making of body fat and, instead, uses it to produce body heat, a process sometimes called *metabolic thermogenesis*.[17] In short, both processes resulting from a low-protein diet—increased thermogenesis and increased physical activity—divert calories away from the making of body fat. In these and other studies, the key difference critical to body weight loss or gain is the *way* that calories are used by the body, not the *amount* of calories consumed.

This doesn't just happen to rats; the results of these laboratory animal studies proved consistent with our observations on humans in rural China. Calorie consumption per unit of body weight in China was significantly higher than that of Westerners,[18,19] yet China's body mass index (BMI) was substantially lower.

To use lay language, the Chinese people in the study consumed more calories but weighed less—even after compensating for their greater physical activity. Like our experimental animals, these people were eating a diet low in protein (but very high in carbohydrates!), almost all of which was provided by plant-based foods. Based on previous findings by a group of British researchers,[20] it's reasonable to assume that these people were turning the consumed calories to body heat during physical activity, just like our experimental animals. (I see this rather like the feeling of sluggishness one gets after consuming a high-fat, high-protein meal, as opposed to the energetic "light" feeling after a low-protein, low-fat meal.) Remember, too, that only a very small shift in the body's distribution of calories (50 per day) can make an important difference in body weight even in one year.

What our findings in China suggest, then, is that consuming a whole food, plant-based, high-carbohydrate diet (in which 75 to 80 percent of total energy comes from plants) minimizes weight gain by shifting the distribution of energy to physical activity and the production of body heat rather than long-term storage as fat. Weight gain, it turns out, has little or nothing to do with the number of calories we consume and everything to do with the way those calories are used in the body.

### Research (Out of) Context

These sometimes puzzling, provocative, and difficult-to-follow findings should prompt questions as to the reliability of the evidence. Taubes cites hundreds of studies to "prove" his theories. But I maintain that his conclusions—chiefly, that low-fat diets make people fat—are patently unsupported by both the historical and scientific evidence. How can I say that? The answer to this question lies in a consideration of the way research is typically done, as well as the way scientists, and Taubes and I here specifically, interpret the findings.

Taubes uses evidence from narrowly defined studies within a very complex body of evidence to create a new narrative of his own making. When isolated facts like these are knitted together, the risk that the narrative can be influenced by personal bias is higher, especially when the final product is not subjected to and/or supported by professional evaluation and scrutiny. And Taubes' work has never been evaluated by professional, qualified peers.

In Taubes' case, there is also something more to consider: none of the research studies he cites are his. He is not a scientist and has conducted no experimental research of his own. All of this heightens the likelihood that the narrative he has constructed from these disparate details has been impacted by his already formed prejudices. While research scientists are not immune to bias (indeed, as I describe in *Whole*, certain types of bias are endemic in the scientific community), the fact that they have to contend with the results of their own research, and can't pretend to ignore them, limits to some extent their leeway to "cherry pick" facts the way Taubes has.

The way Taubes has chosen what evidence to include is a bit like the results of a prosecuting attorney having sole authority over jury selection. The jurors would likely all be honorable citizens, but they would almost certainly represent a specific slice of the total population, with characteristics and outlooks that favor the case for the prosecution.

Each of the papers Taubes references, therefore, deserves a careful examination based on a number of important issues:

- the many experimental factors and conditions that may have impacted the paper's results;
- the appropriateness of the experimental study design;
- the level of statistical significance;
- the source of funding, not just for each particular study but for its authors in general;
- the professional reputation of the journal; and
- the method used for interpreting the data.

These issues are not easy to evaluate for most readers, who are not likely to be familiar with scientific research protocol. Indeed, these issues are not always easy to evaluate for experienced researchers either, especially when the researchers are not working in the immediate field of study.

I confess that I have not obtained all of Taubes' references for my own critical review and interpretation—a task made unusually difficult by his cumbersome and questionable method of referencing.[21] Thus, for expediency, I have chosen to extend to Taubes the courtesy of simply accepting, as is, the evidence (often indirect) that he believes supports the health value of the low-carb diet (lower body weight, less incidence of diabetes, etc.).

However, even if we assume the evidence to be equally valid, a problem remains: To explain the results of the studies that support the low-carb diet—the decreases in body weight, blood lipids, and, importantly, circulating insulin when initially following a low-carb diet versus the Standard American Diet (SAD)—Taubes must weave together details that, while they individually may be sound, do not accurately describe the function of the whole.

First we need to review some basics that Taubes uses in those conclusions—details about the body's function when it comes to carbohydrates that are generally accepted as true but are in fact far from it. Though Taubes begins in the right place, his is a very narrow view of the results of energy production and metabolism as it interacts with countless other events inside the body.

When carbohydrates are consumed and the food is digested in the intestine, glucose is produced. This glucose is absorbed into the bloodstream and then, assisted by the hormone insulin, enters cells, where it is oxidized to produce energy. This satisfies our hunger—the need for energy that arises in cells and is translated to us as the desire to eat food.

Glucose not used to produce energy immediately may be stored in the liver and muscles as glycogen, a starch-like polysaccharide; it, too, is available for use by cells rather quickly, when energy is needed. There is also a second option for unused glucose: it may be converted to triglyceride (fat), a more stable storage form of energy that gradually accumulates to form adipose tissue, the stuff of obesity.[22]

After consuming a meal, the body's blood glucose level rises, then returns to baseline within a few hours as the glucose is either used by cells to provide immediate energy or converted for storage. Both glucose and insulin blood levels rise and fall together in waves as we intermittently consume meals because glucose entering the bloodstream automatically triggers insulin's release. All of this is a very normal process in healthy people.

For too many people, however, a diet high in refined carbohydrates and simple sugars results in consistently elevated glucose levels in the bloodstream. To compensate, these high glucose levels require a continuously high level of insulin that, for some as yet unknown reason, gradually loses its ability to facilitate glucose's entry into cells. To overcome this diminished insulin activity—or "insulin resistance"—the pancreas responds by secreting still more insulin, thereby creating a vicious cycle with adverse consequences. Higher blood sugar levels lead to the release of more insulin and, if this state is prolonged, more insulin resistance, which leads to higher blood sugar levels. We might therefore consider the effects of this cycle a disease of insulin excess or, perhaps, glucose toxicity, as seen in Type 2 diabetes, obesity, and heart disease. The reason this happens, according to Taubes, is the regular overconsumption of carbohydrates.

Insulin has many other normal functions besides assisting in the cellular entry and metabolism of glucose. It also may assist in the uptake, metabolism, and storage of glucose as triglycerides (fat). Although this stored fat can be recalled and metabolized to produce energy, a high level of insulin in the bloodstream tends to block this conversion of stored fat back to energy. An overabundance of insulin therefore leaves cells elsewhere in the body hungry for energy. In response, we continue to eat—and continue to gain weight, as the body stores more glucose.

According to Taubes, the most practical solution to this problem of too much insulin in the blood is to reduce the demand for insulin by not flooding the system with high-glucose foods, especially those refined carbohydrates that are readily digested and absorbed and often produce fat.

There are a few things wrong with this, even on the surface. Although the fundamentals of this story about carbohydrate digestion, absorption, and utilization are essentially correct, it should be noted that it mostly refers to the effects of *refined* carbohydrates, not total carbohydrates, which are found in whole foods. In addition, the result of short-term, out-of-context findings—those obtained in the test tube, so to speak—must be reconciled with long-term health outcomes. There are many examples where a laboratory-based, out-of-context finding does not equate with a true-life experience. (Perhaps one of the better-known examples concerns the antioxidant beta-carotene, the proper form of vitamin A, which when present in food is associated with a healthy response but when consumed as a supplement causes an unhealthy response.)

I repeat: parts of what Taubes says here are definitely accurate, to the best of current scientific knowledge, and the findings he uses to construct this story may represent high-quality research. But the story itself, as well as the solution he comes to (the low-carb diet), is just not true; evidence from many other studies shows that high carbohydrate, as in the whole food, plant-based diet, also can produce fat degradation and loss of body fat. The research findings Taubes uses refer to events that have been isolated from their natural environments.

The process of combining isolated events into a cohesive story only works if the pieces of the puzzle are put into the right places. Sadly, this same process can just as easily be used to prove something that is in fact untrue. For example, if we wanted to prove that Coca-Cola promotes health, we could construct a study in which some people were given Coca-Cola to drink, while others were not given any liquid at all—and never look at the effects of Coca-Cola compared to water. This is the dilemma with almost all diet and health research: whether we have enough or the right kind of details assembled to reliably create a hypothesis that really works.

I'm not suggesting that all research looking at specific details (research that is characteristically reductionist in nature) is purposefully biased or of no value. Well-constructed reductionist studies can be used to deepen our understanding of the whole of human health by providing explanations—specific details and mechanisms—that stabilize and sustain wholistic research: research that looks not just at the evidence from one study, but at all the evidence currently available, and draws conclusions accordingly. Reductionist research must be conducted in the service of "big picture" truths that can be gleaned only from a wholistic look at reality. And this is especially true for nutrition studies.

A classic metaphor, which I explore in detail in *Whole*, is the old story of six blind men tasked with describing an elephant. One feels the trunk and describes the elephant as a hose. Another feels the tusk and describes a spear, a third apprehends the leg as a pillar, and so on. All of their explorations have merit, but each individual's conclusions leads to an erroneous understanding of the thing the group has been tasked with describing. Only when the starting point is an understanding of the whole elephant can we make sense of the separate findings.

Any study that looks at only one disease, one nutrient, or one population out of context and contradicts all the wholistic evidence cannot be seen, on its own, as proof. When a reductionist finding contradicts the big picture, it doesn't make sense to tear down that big picture. Rather, we look for exceptions, nuances, and deeper understandings—ways of reconciling an outlier data point with the demonstrated reality. Sometimes we find that the conflicting detail is a fluke (a random result of statistical uncertainty) when we repeat the experiment and fail to replicate it. Sometimes we discover that the premise of the experiment itself is flawed.

Rarely do unexplained data points bring down entire structures of thought, though it does happen on occasion; we call this phenomenon a paradigm shift. For example, Copernicus and Galileo discovered outlier data that ultimately invalidated the entire earth-centric system of astronomy that had been common knowledge since ancient times. But we can't look at a single reductionist finding that conflicts with current theory and summarily declare the theory null and void. Outlying and contradictory data must be honored, but we honor them by following them on a rigorous search for truth, not by elevating them to dogma simply because doing so enhances our pocketbooks or our egos.

This, in essence, is what the low-carb advocates are doing. By ignoring findings that comprehensively describe the whole, they elevate outlying or contradictory data to dogma.

## How Low in Fat Is "Low-Fat"?

There's one more significant way in which Taubes gets things wrong, and it has to do with a failure of definition around the term "low fat." In fact, the misuse of their term "low fat" by the low-carb advocates is one of the most egregious misrepresentations in their entire narrative.

The low-carb-advocates' argument in favor of a low-carb (but high-fat!) diet rests on their mistaken idea that increased dietary fat doesn't matter—that dieters have been diligently pursuing the government's low-fat recommendations for years, and yet no one's getting any thinner or healthier. In fact, low-carb advocates claim, these government-recommended low-fat diets in effect *cause* obesity.

These pronouncements rest on the assumption that those "low-fat" dieters are *actually following a low-fat diet*. But this is simply not the case. It's a myth. This so-called low-fat diet is anything but low in fat.

According to Taubes in *Good Calories, Bad Calories*, the inflection point tipping the nation's scales toward a low-fat diet was the published research of University of Minnesota professor Ancel Keys in the 1950s on the connection between dietary fat and heart disease. Keys was a well-known nutritional authority prior to this work; the K-rations of World War II were formulated by and named for him. He was also known for his "starvation studies," in which he subjected conscientious objector volunteers to near-starvation conditions to discover the effects of nutritional deprivation on human physiology.

Keys began his post-war research because of an anomalous finding: the wealthiest businessmen in Minnesota, who presumably could afford the best food and health care, were suffering a disproportionately high rate of heart disease. Keys' intellectual pursuits had all been about starvation and the minimum calories needed by soldiers in battle conditions, so you can imagine his surprise to discover that a surfeit of rich animal foods—which were then thought to be, as they still are by most today, the highest-quality foods—appeared to make men less healthy rather than more so.

Keys' subsequent research suggested a link between diets high in total fat, especially saturated fat and cholesterol, and heart disease. His first studies looked at Minnesota businessmen, and he later broadened his research to seven countries in four regions of the world. This Seven Countries Study[23,24] published as an article in 1970 and as a book in 1980, caused quite a stir among public officials and politicians who were concerned with national health policy. In later studies, Keys broadened the scope of his research and discovered a similar effect of dietary fat on obesity, diabetes, and cancer.

According to Keys, promotion of these diseases by high-fat diets could be explained by the fact that fats, at 9 calories/gram, are calorie dense, as opposed to carbohydrate and protein, which have 4 calories/gram. High-fat diets therefore meant calorie-dense diets and more calorie consumption. This was a convenient way to combine two ideas that were popular at the time—that calories and fat each increased obesity and obesity-related diseases—into one.

Keys' focus on fat, especially saturated fat and cholesterol, implied that consumption of foods rich in these nutrients, especially meat and eggs, should be curbed. The widespread popularity of his research also resulted in a shift in the marketplace away from the fat content of cow's milk to low-fat and even skim milk. (On the dairy farm where I grew up, we valued milk for its butterfat content, both in the pricing of the finished milk and in the breeding programs designed to produce offspring capable of producing high-fat milk. I recall when we got word down on the farm that public opinion was moving away from high-fat milk. It was Ancel Keys' research findings that caused the shift.)

Keys vigorously promoted his research findings, publishing two popular diet books with his wife, Margaret, (*Eat Well and Stay Well* [1963] and *How to Eat Well and Stay Well the Mediterranean Way* [1975]), alongside his scholarly work. A typical sentiment from Keys: North Americans make "the stomach the garbage disposal unit for a long list of harmful foods."[25]

I had the privilege to meet Keys twice: once when he lectured at Cornell while I was a graduate student and much later when Keys, then in his nineties, was in attendance at a lecture I gave at Harvard on my research findings in China. Keys' ultimate contribution to the field of nutrition may have been the example he set by "walking his talk"—he died in 2004, just two months shy of his 101st birthday!

Taubes claims that it was Keys, more than any other writer or researcher, who focused public attention on dietary fat as the main culprit for obesity and poor health. According to Taubes, U.S. government policy based on Keys' research not only failed to improve our health, it also caused the very epidemics (obesity, cardiovascular disease, diabetes) that it was trying to prevent.

This interpretation is incorrect on two levels. First, Taubes assumes that Keys advocated lower consumption of saturated fat and cholesterol as the *only* strategy for reducing heart disease. While this is partly true, Keys was also concerned with the source of these nutrients: that is, animal-based foods. For example, he wrote while discussing the very high correlation of saturated fat with serum cholesterol in population-based studies and the "distress [it caused in] the dairy and meat industries" that these industries' "products account for almost all of the saturated fat in Britain and the United States, and most other countries."[26] Second, to my knowledge, Keys never really defined his recommended "low-fat diet" in terms of an ideal percentage of calories from fat; he thought that relying on specific benchmarks set by policy makers did not make sense.[27]

In other words, while getting some of the details right, Taubes misses the nuance of this history by falsely representing the definition of a low-fat diet as well as its alleged health effects.

The very lowest level of dietary fat ever advocated by a federally funded report (one I coauthored, and the recommendations of which I was, regrettably, unable to influence as much as I would have liked) was 30 percent of daily calories.[28] By no stretch of the imagination can this be considered "low fat." A 1999 national survey showed that average dietary fat intake never dropped down to this level, at best reaching about 33 percent of total calories.[29] The idea that a government recommendation to reduce dietary fat to 30 percent or lower was ever reached, or that such a level would be sufficient to demonstrate a decrease in disease, is ludicrous. It's akin to telling smokers to cut down from five packs a day to four and a half—and then, upon seeing no results, claiming that decreased smoking doesn't make a difference and is not worth pursuing.

Not only were the "low-fat" recommendations from this report and other sources never heeded, but the absolute intake of fat did not decrease. As a nation, we may have flirted with the idea of a low-fat diet, but we never actually succeeded in following such recommendations. While we may have reduced the percentage of our dietary fat over the last few decades (albeit slowly), because our total food intake (and calories) has gone up, dietary fat consumption, if anything, has *increased*.[30] The suggestion that we have adhered to that 30 percent recommendation and, further, that having done so, we failed to achieve the expected health results, is fantasy. The argument by Taubes and his advocates that low-fat diets have not decreased obesity, and perhaps have even caused it, is a straw man fallacy.

To be fair to Taubes, there was a lot of focus in the scientific and health community on the evils of fat from the 1950s to the 1970s. But he and other low-carb advocates underemphasize the shift in this focus on fat, both in the health community and in public policy, that began with the 1977 McGovern Committee and the 1982 report on diet, nutrition, and cancer (the report I reference above, which proposed the lowest recommendations of calories from fat). In that report, we indicated that fat was not the main cause of cancer and other diseases, but rather a marker of the dietary proportion of (naturally low in fat) plant-based foods to (naturally high in fat) animal-based foods. In other words, a diet truly low in fat (e.g., 10 percent of calories) is by definition a diet high in good quality whole (not processed) plant-based foods and low in animal-based foods.

The McGovern report's recommendations on dietary fat were meant to be understood in the context of the overall goal: to increase the consumption of plant-based foods while decreasing the consumption of animal-based foods. I'm confident Taubes knows this; it's stated explicitly in the report, in the comments especially on the consumption of meat. Yet he still focuses his arguments on dietary fat and the failure of the (incorrectly labeled) low-fat diet, while ignoring the main issue: the balance of animal- and plant-based foods.

THE MCGOVERN REPORT

Let's take a closer look at the history of the McGovern Committee report on the association of dietary fat with heart disease: both what it really said and what impact it really had. McGovern's highly political committee was first formed in the early 1970s, after McGovern's failed presidential bid and after his visit to the Pritikin health clinic, where he witnessed firsthand the dramatic health benefits of consuming a diet very different from the one he and most Americans followed: one truly low in fat and high in whole plant-based foods. After inviting expert testimony, the McGovern Committee recommended that dietary fat, especially saturated fat and cholesterol, be decreased, as Keys and other researchers had suggested. Because this kind of fat is far more plentiful in animal-based foods, the McGovern Committee therefore recommended reducing the consumption of meat[31] as well as the consumption of "butterfat, eggs, and other cholesterol sources." Unfortunately, the marketplace did not respond by changing the proportions of plant- and animal-based foods. Instead, politicians, marketers, and consumers alike focused specifically, and inaccurately, on the modification of their fat intake.

A preliminary 1976 recommendation by the McGovern Committee to cut back on meat consumption in general created a furor among politicians and the electorate alike. As a result, the committee revised their report in 1977 to recommend a decrease in red meat consumption but not the white meat of fish and chicken[32]—a political decision, not a scientific one. Even that did not prove enough of a political compromise, however. McGovern personally told me that several prominent Midwest senators subsequently lost their 1980 elections because their support for his committee's recommendations upset their political base of livestock farmers. Professor Mark Hegsted, who was on leave from Harvard University and acting as a full-time expert consultant to the McGovern Committee staff, told me several stories about exceptionally hostile reactions from certain groups to these plant-focused recommendations. Even though the McGovern report only concerned the effect of diet on cardiovascular disease, the public furor—or that of the lobbyists, anyway—was intense. I remember wondering at the time what kind of adverse reaction might occur were there to be a similar focus on dietary effects on cancer, the much more feared disease.

Shortly thereafter, a U.S. Senate Committee wondered the same thing. They organized a public hearing and asked the director of the National Cancer Institute (NCI), Vince DeVita, for testimony. During that testimony, DeVita said that he could not be sure if the McGovern Committee's recommendations about the effects of diet on heart disease would similarly apply to the effects of diet on cancer.[33] Hearing this, the Senate Committee appropriated about $1 million for the NCI to organize an expert committee at the NAS to review the existing literature on the topic. I was invited, along with twelve others, to be on this committee, which eventually produced the landmark 1982 NAS report on diet, nutrition, and cancer.[34] Although we recommended reducing dietary fat to 30 percent or less of total dietary calories—a level similar to that in the McGovern report on heart disease—we also suggested, as a goal (versus the more proactive "recommendation"), the increased consumption of whole foods such as fruits, vegetables, and grains.

As expected, the release of this report fanned the flames of public discussion about food and health. According to the NAS, it was the most sought-after report in their history. I appeared on the PBS show *McNeil-Lehrer News Hour* and was featured in *People*, among many other magazines, to discuss the report. And, as with the McGovern Committee report, political fallout was intense. A prominent task force of the agricultural industry, the Council for Agricultural Science and Technology (CAST),[35] quickly responded; within two weeks, they had published a very critical commentary of our report and placed copies of it on the desk of every congressperson and senator. A few of us testified to congressional committees about it.

Our goal (not a recommendation) in the NAS report[36] to reduce dietary fat to 30 percent or less was not merely an attempt to mimic the McGovern Committee's similar recommendation. It was intended to emphasize the dietary change that we thought worth pursuing for cancer control, based on the available evidence at that time. We stated in our executive summary that the evidence on cancer suggested an ideal diet considerably *lower* in total fat than our 30 percent goal—perhaps 20 percent of calories or lower—which would put even more emphasis on naturally low-fat whole plant-based foods. We chose the arbitrary and more conservative benchmark of 30 percent because going lower might have suggested a decrease in consumption of protein, especially animal-based protein, and politicians then, as now, were sensitive to the interests of dairy and livestock organizations.

The 30 percent dietary fat goal was not intended to single out fat or any other nutrient as the specific and only dietary effector of cancer. The report heavily emphasized the consumption of whole foods, especially fruits, vegetables, and grains. In doing so, we clearly stated that none of our specific goals applied to individual nutrients, such as adding individual micronutrients in supplement form or subtracting fat.

As marketplace events developed, however, considerable emphasis was given to individual nutrients such as fat (eat less), fiber (eat more), and vitamins and minerals (take supplements). These and other similar responses have been the source of one of my greatest frustrations regarding the way science is interpreted and communicated to the general public. It seems that whenever whole plant-based foods are brought up for discussion, the conversation turns in some way to the exploitation of single nutrients, whether they are fat, carbohydrates, protein, or vitamin and mineral supplements. That's where the money was and still is.

Still, recommendations during the 1980s and 1990s by respected institutions to increase consumption of plant-based foods continued to be published,[37,38] leading up to the 1997 World Cancer Research Fund/American Institute for Cancer Research report,[39] which I co-chaired. The first recommendation of this 1997 report bluntly stated: "Consume a plant-based diet."

In *Good Calories, Bad Calories*, Taubes grossly oversimplifies and distorts the history of the diet and health field. He makes it seem as if the entire field is focused only on dietary fat as an evil nutrient and, further, that scientists found a dietary level of 30 percent fat to be sufficiently "low." Rather, the most important message surfacing during the period from the 1970s to the 1990s was to increase consumption of whole plant-based foods and, by inference, to decrease consumption of animal-based foods.

Taubes, unfortunately, is not the only one who missed that message; most of the public did, too.

# THE OPTIMAL HUMAN DIET FOR IDEAL WEIGHT, VIBRANT HEALTH, AND LONGEVITY

Good science tells us the optimal way to eat is what I call the Whole Food, Plant-Based (WFPB) diet. This is something the evidence had been clear on long before I was considering my lab's own experimental findings. Many decades earlier, everyone was regularly advised, if vaguely, to "eat more fruits and vegetables." But this may be the first time you've encountered this much evidence for the remarkable health-promoting effects of a WFPB diet. Not because the idea is "fringe" or the evidence is weak; rather, because the food, medical, and pharmaceutical industries have a lot to lose if our society wises up to the health-giving properties of whole, plant-based foods and the disease-causing properties of animal-based and highly processed foods. The evidence points clearly to a WFPB diet as the one that can most reliably deliver radiant long-term health, as well as the slim bodies we desire.

First, a definition. The WFPB diet consists of whole foods—that is, foods as close to their natural state as possible. A wide variety of fruits, vegetables, grains, nuts, and seeds make up the bulk of the diet. It includes no refined products, such as white sugar or white flour; no additives, preservatives, or other chemical concoctions, which our bodies were never programmed to recognize or digest; no refined fats, including olive or coconut oils; and minimal—or, better yet, no—consumption of animal products, perhaps 0 to 5 percent of total calories at most.

By consuming a broad range of plant foods, we don't really have to worry about the specifics of calories, carbohydrates, fats, protein, or even vitamins; the numbers more or less take care of themselves. Since plant foods are largely carbohydrate based, the percentages of calories tend to approach 80 percent from carbohydrates, 10 percent from protein, and 10 percent from fat. Of course, if you continually binge on avocados and nuts and avoid leafy greens, you can distort the spirit of the diet. But even with your best efforts, you'd be hard-pressed to reach even as much as 15 percent of your total calories from protein with a WFPB diet.

Could you just increase your consumption of total protein from animal sources and still get the desired benefits of a WFPB diet? Yes, but getting 15 percent of your calories from plant protein is not the same as getting 15 percent of your calories from animal protein, at least in part because of the major difference such a change would make in the consumption of *other* nutrients that accompany animal-based foods.

In my first book, *The China Study: The Most Comprehensive Study of Nutrition Ever Conducted and the Startling Implications for Diet, Weight Loss, and Long-Term Health* (2004), which I coauthored with my son Tom, I shared the research that my lab and many other scientists had accumulated to demonstrate the remarkable health effects of the WFPB diet. In my second book, *Whole*, I discuss why this evidence is more reliable and accurate than the science that supposedly supports high-animal-foods diets. For the full story, I recommend those books. For our purposes here, I'll give you the short version.

As summarized in *The China Study*, the WFPB diet provides an exceptionally rich bonanza of antioxidants, complex carbohydrates, and optimum intakes of fat, protein, vitamins, and minerals, many of which contribute to disease prevention. Any deviation from this model—as with consuming animal-based or processed foods—causes you to miss out on the vast benefits of these life-sustaining nutrients. For the most part, supplementation and fortification with individual nutrients or combinations thereof will not restore what whole foods can do for health.

Moreover, and very much to the point for this book, the "high-carb" WFPB diet decreases the risk of obesity-related degenerative diseases—in direct opposition to what Taubes' model of sharply reduced carbohydrate consumption predicts.

## *Effects on Glucose: The WFPB Diet Versus the Low-Carb Diet*

As you'll recall, Taubes' model states that a low-carb, high-animal-protein diet will reduce blood glucose, insulin, and cholesterol, thus decreasing the risk for obesity, diabetes, and heart disease. But many reports show, in various ways, that the opposite is true.

My friend David Kritchevsky, who was probably the leading researcher in this area until his death, found[40] that "protein of animal origin is more cholesterolemic [leading to higher cholesterol in the bloodstream] and atherogenic [contributing to heart disease] than protein of plant origin for rabbits," citing several studies[41]—a distinction between types of protein that was first noted in regard to atherosclerosis more than sixty years ago.[42] He found the same to be true for humans, as well.[43] We observed a similar distinction between soy and casein protein (the principle protein in milk) in my lab when they were compared in our studies on experimental cancer with rats.[44]

Likewise, animal and plant protein have completely different effects on insulin. Dr. Richard Hubbard of the Loma Linda School of Medicine and his colleague Albert Sanchez have done significant research on the effects of plant- and animal-based proteins,[45] on findings that directly concern Taubes' model.

According to their research, plant protein actually *decreases* insulin and *increases* glucagon (the counterweight to insulin), preventing or reversing diabetes. A higher plant protein/animal protein ratio represses the formation of fat (triglycerides), while reducing the activity of a key enzyme in the synthesis of cholesterol. In short, the persistently low insulin levels commonly observed with plant protein–based diets (as with the WFPB diet—though not, importantly, with diets high in *refined* carbohydrates) are associated with persistently low blood cholesterol levels, among other biomarkers of diseases like heart disease, obesity, many cancers, and other serious ailments that track together in populations.

What this means is that the high-carb, plant protein–based WFPB diet behaves *exactly the opposite* of how Taubes predicts it will. Taubes says that a high-carb diet increases insulin, which converts the high blood sugar to fat and then represses the conversion of the fat back to energy, leaving fat stored in the cells—and this is why people get fat and eventually suffer from diabetes and other diseases associated with obesity. Although this may sound attractive and may be true for people consuming a diet high in *refined* carbohydrates (i.e., sugar), there is no evidence that this applies to a WFPB[46,47,48] diet that is high in total carbohydrate and low in protein, all of which is plant based. Virtually every person who uses the WFPB diet loses weight, reduces their blood sugar and insulin levels, and resolves diabetes and related diseases. A plant protein–based diet (as in the high-carb WFPB diet) also decreases total blood cholesterol and the formation of plaques that lead to heart disease, effects not seen from a low-carb, animal protein–based diet. In direct refutation of Taubes' predictions, the WFPB diet also successfully promotes weight loss, and it does so without the serious side effects that accompany the low-carb diet.

I summarized the side effects of the low-carb diet earlier: more headaches, bad breath, constipation, and muscle cramps. The low-carb diet shows little or no consistent health benefits when compared with other diet strategies, which are free of these side effects. And if apparent benefits do occur on the low-carb diet—weight loss, in particular—they are not sustained. In addition to being both inconsistent and relatively small, the alleged health benefits tend to disappear within a year.[49] But more to the point, the low-carb diet's ability to show *any* benefit depends on the control diet against which it is compared.

### Low-Carb Diet "Benefits" in Context

Usually the low-carb diet is evaluated by comparing it to the Standard American Diet (SAD)—which, as we've seen, is misleadingly labeled "low fat" when in reality (and compared to the WFPB diet, in which only 10 percent of the calories come from fat) it's *high* in fat, as well as high in animal protein and low in antioxidants and complex carbohydrates. About 30 to 40 percent of the SAD's calories come from fat. This is a huge difference! The SAD is also, on average, about 70 percent higher in total protein than the amount recommended and easily provided by a WFPB diet (meaning that the protein consumption of about half of Americans is even higher than that). Almost all of this excess protein is from animal-based foods. To put it another way: at least 90 to 95 percent of Americans are consuming a carbohydrate-poor, relatively rich diet that is already near Atkins levels in its inclusion of animal protein.

Because of this similarity, when an Atkins/Taubes low-carb diet is compared with modest variations of the SAD, any observed beneficial effects are mostly random and relatively trivial, though that doesn't prevent the low-carb spin masters from making them into headlines whenever possible. A true dietary comparison, by contrast, would also include the WFPB diet—but this almost never happens.

Nowhere is this more clear than in a 2007 study by Gardner et al.[50] The study's objective was to compare the ability of four popular diets to reduce body weight, and their particular focus was on investigating if low-fat diets were actually able to reduce body weight. Therefore, the flaw that I found especially repugnant—and obvious—was their failure to use a truly "low-fat" diet for comparison: they compared the results of Atkins and several other diets to what they *claimed* was the Ornish diet (a low fat, whole plant food diet based on the work of Dr. Dean Ornish, a pioneer in the use of a WFPB diet to reverse heart disease).

The true Ornish Diet, like the WFPB diet, contains only 10 to 12 percent fat. But the authors of this Atkins-friendly research paper instead used a grossly distorted version of the Ornish Diet, one that contained *29 percent fat*, and called it "extremely low fat"! The distortion was even more serious because the authors' so-called Ornish Diet also contained 18 percent protein, which is 70 to 80 percent higher than the amount generally present in plant-based diets. In the Gardner et al fabricated Ornish Diet, fat and protein comprised 48 percent of total calories, rather than the 20 to 22 percent in the true Ornish plan.

The other diets used for comparison were two very similar variations on the SAD: the LEARN[51] and Zone[52] diets. Together, these four nutritionally similar diets were severely limited in their ability to show meaningful and statistically significant differences, due to their similarities in dietary fat and protein (the two measures that best represent the differences between these plans and a truly low-fat, low-protein, WFPB diet): fat and protein accounted for 65, 54, 51, and 48 percent of total calories, respectively, which are all far in excess of the WFPB diet's 22 percent. Of course, there was one scientifically random difference observed at the end of the study: they found a slightly lower body weight for the Atkins Diet than the SAD and Ornish Diets, and this scientifically nonsignificant finding made headlines as if it were extremely important.

Because this study was destined to create major media attention, it required critique at the time it was published in the acclaimed *Journal of the Medical Association* (JAMA). Critique in conventional science generally occurs in the widely accepted letters-to-the-editor format, which might be considered another aspect of the peer-review process. Four of us in the profession therefore duly submitted our letters to the journal editor to point out the study's serious flaws and seek the investigators' responses. Usually such letters are published after some modest peer review—but not in this case. The JAMA editor denied all four of our critique letters, including one letter from Dr. Ornish himself, the man whose diet was being so grossly misrepresented. Over the course of my career, I have published many research papers and served on several science journal editorial review boards, and never have I witnessed such unprincipled and unsavory behavior. Readers had a right to hear both our critiques and the researchers' responses to them, but instead they heard nothing. And so this study, like many similar findings, went unchallenged and has since been asserted as foundational evidence proving the superiority of the low-carb diet.

Another recent and highly publicized study also failed to include diets of sufficient nutrient difference that would have enabled the researchers to analyze and discern their effects and thus evaluate and understand the different diets in their proper context. The study, "Primary Prevention of Cardiovascular Disease with a Mediterranean Diet,"[53] published in the *New England Journal of Medicine*, concerned the supposed health benefits of the Mediterranean diet in regards to heart attack and stroke. Its participants, who were all at high cardiovascular risk but did not have cardiovascular disease at the time of the study, were randomly assigned to one of three diets: "a Mediterranean diet supplemented with extra-virgin olive oil, a Mediterranean diet supplemented with mixed nuts, or a control diet (advice to reduce dietary fat)."

According to the researchers, their findings showed that both versions of the Mediterranean diet—the one with added olive oil and the one with added nuts—were healthier than a standard low-fat American diet. The "low fat" group suffered 109 "events" (strokes and heart attacks), compared to just 96 for the Mediterranean olive oil group and 83 for the Mediterranean nuts group.

At first glance, you might agree with the researchers (and the low-carb hucksters) who called this finding a major blow in the battle against misguided low-fat dieting. But diving a little deeper into this research reveals something very different.

Before I tell you the actual numbers reported by the researchers, take a wild guess at the percentages of fat in the three diets. You'd think that a diet described as "low fat" would include a lot less fat than those touted as "low carb," right? Well, you'd be wrong.[54] By the end of the trial, the two Mediterranean diet groups were getting a little more than 41 percent of their calories from fat, while the so-called "low fat" control group was getting 37 percent of their calories from fat.

Thirty-seven percent of total calories from dietary fat is considered a low-fat diet? Four percent is a significant difference in dietary fat consumption?

Just for fun, let's graph these results and compare them to SAD and WFPB diets:

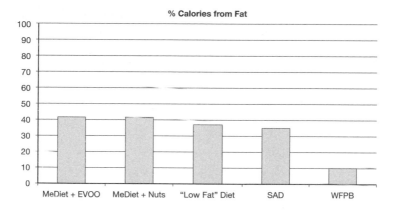

Here's what the headlines should have read: "Three almost identically bad diets produce almost identically bad health outcomes."

I cannot overstate the seriousness of this distortion of what constitutes a low-fat diet, or how common this distortion appears in scientific papers published by low-carb advocates. There have been three relatively recent reviews of the low-carb diet as compared with other diets, published in 2003,[55] 2006,[56] and 2009,[57] respectively. These summaries are quite repetitive, mostly including the same research studies, in which the subjects are generally overweight to obese. Each report concludes that, on average, low-carb-diet interventions generally result in some weight loss and favorable but variable changes in indicators of cardiovascular disease risk (conclusions that are highlighted in the abstracts, which provide the main and only information from these studies that most laypeople will see). And throughout this literature, we see the same misinterpretation of a "low-fat" diet and the same lack of diversity across diets repeated ad nauseum. "Low fat" is always approximately 30 percent fat (or higher), not the WFPB diet's 10 to 12 percent fat. In these studies, both the control diet and the low-carb diet are high in animal protein and low in plant-based foods, making it very difficult to see the results we know exist when a much wider range of nutritional compositions are available for comparison.

## THE WHOLE TRUTH ABOUT LOW-CARB

Low-carb advocates have succeeded in winning over a substantial segment of the market for about four decades now. In part, they have done so because their message is one that many people want to hear: good things about their bad habits.

Over the years, I have found it increasingly difficult to accept low-carb advocates' antics. They've changed the benchmark for the definition of a "low-fat" diet and seemed normal. The consumption of high amounts of animal protein. They've used the concept of "low-carb" to negatively reflect on the source of carbs: whole, plant-based foods. And they've done these things for their own self-serving interests: protecting and even expanding the marketing horizon for high-fat, animal protein–based foods.

Taubes and many other low-carb advocates use an abundance of carefully selected but out-of-context details to add a scientific patina to their arguments, which just don't hold up under careful scrutiny. Please don't get me wrong: such details can be, and are, useful when they are employed to describe an accurate whole. But when details are spun into a false narrative to support a diet with unpleasant side effects and serious long-term consequences, it's time to sound the alarm, loud and clear.

When describing their diet, either in research or in general discussion, low-carb advocates usually compare it to our already poor Standard American Diet (SAD) and/or the only slightly modified "low-fat" version recommended by the government. As we've seen, this is a false comparison. Our diet or even its slightly modified government-sanctioned version is not what the low-carb people claim it is. First, the SAD is already high in total protein—about 70 percent higher than ideal—and around 70 percent of it is protein from animal-based foods (thus limiting consumption of plant-based foods and their antioxidants and complex carbohydrates). Second, the SAD contains three to four times the amount of fat the science recommends. In short, it is a fat-rich, protein-rich, and often refined carbohydrate–rich diet. This is the benchmark that's called "low fat" by the low-carb advocates, and this is what they use to prove their diet's superiority over all other types of eating. These are very serious misrepresentations.

To say that the government-recommended "low-fat" diet adopted during the past four decades has only led to more obesity is hubris squared. Even if the American public *had* followed the recommendations and reduced their dietary fat (and the most one could say, in that case, was that dietary fat was reduced from about 35 to 33 percent of total calories), that cannot be used to properly evaluate the health benefits of a truly low-fat diet like the WFPB diet, in which only 10 to 12 percent of calories come from fat.

I am confident that low-carb advocates like Taubes know all this. But rather than allow this to expose their argument for the embarrassment it is, they try to explain these facts away by pejoratively describing the WFPB diet (as with the Ornish Diet in Gardner et al.[58]) as "extreme." Actual low-fat diets are almost never taken into account in these discussions, and when they are, they are distorted to make them more similar to the SAD. In so doing, low-carb advocates cleverly remove the possibility of experimentally observing the real, life-and-death differences between these diets.

Low-carb advocates also focus on weight—not on health. The low-carb diet cannot reverse and sustain the reversal of advanced diseases like the WFPB diet can. When the dietary practices in different countries are compared, high-fat, high-protein diets (like the low-carb diet) are consistently associated with higher, not lower, rates of several cancers, heart disease, and other diseases. Plant-based diets show the opposite effect. In fact, I do not know of a single study among the hundreds undertaken where it has been shown that a low-carb (high-protein, high-fat, low-fiber/complex carbohydrate) diet is associated with less cancer, heart disease, or diabetes.

Perhaps the most telling report on the low-carb diet and health is the recent summary of 17 studies published in January 2013 involving 272,216 subjects,[59] in which a low-carb diet showed a statistically significant *31 percent increase* in total deaths. This finding is even more telling than the statistics suggest because this 31 percent increase is in comparison to the *already* high mortality typically observed for the SAD, when compared to a whole food, plant-based diet. Also, this study is the first opportunity for us to consider low-carb claims and inferences based on long-term population-based data from multiple nations. These findings, and the inability of the low-carb diet to reverse serious diseases like heart disease and Type 2 diabetes, makes the initial decreases in body weight often observed with the low-carb diet "irrelevant," as the authors of this report note.

Low-carb advocates like to discount such population-based studies because they do not allow us to determine causality. But this complaint is valid only when made against investigations that have been designed to look for specific, single-nutrient or single-chemical causes of disease. This is not how nutrition works. The dismissal is much less valid when an investigation is looking for associations between broad classes of food—as is the case in these studies, which looked for effects on a broad class of disease outcomes from broad classes of foods that owe their effects to broad classes of nutrients.

The only health claim low-carb advocates make that is worthy of positive note is their warning against refined carbohydrates (refined flours and sugars). But even then, they use this warning largely to try to make a larger point: that all "carbs" are bad. They invented the word "carb" and use it to paint all carbohydrates—all plant-based foods, since these are the sole source of carbohydrates—with the same brush. It's long been documented that refined carbohydrates—carbohydrates that are no longer in their natural, wholistic form—cause health problems. That does not mean that we can use this finding to smear complex carbohydrates, including fiber and starch, in general.

The arguments for the low-carb diet are built entirely from out-of-context, highly reductionist results, woven together into a picture that does not reflect either the summation of scientific data or the reality of health. And that health—not just short-term, unsustainable weight loss, but true, lasting, vibrant health— whether it be for individual people, for entire societies, or for the planet, is the goal to which we all should aspire.

It is time that the low-carb diet, and its alleged benefits, be dismissed as a serious fraud. It is only a continuation of the already poor nutritional status offered by the standard American diet, in a direction that actually makes our individual and collective health worse.

# APPENDIX:
# THE PALEO DIET

In the preceding text, I listed several variations on the low-carb diet, including Mary Dan and Michael Eades' *Protein Power*, Barry Sears' *Enter the Zone*, Peter D'Adamo's *Eat Right 4 Your Type*, Arthur Agatson's *South Beach Diet*, and Eric Westman's *The New Atkins for a New You*. But the version that has been getting the most attention in recent years is *The Paleo Diet*. First published in 2002 and written by Loren Cordain, an exercise physiology professor at Colorado State University, its basic message emphasizing high protein consumption is now offered in dozens of versions and formats, according to Amazon listings. That message, at its core, is low carb. It's especially so by whole food, plant-based diet standards: it allows for, and even encourages, a diet that includes as much as 30 to 50 percent of calories from fat and 30 to 50 percent from protein, leaving only a small amount of calories to be supplied by carbohydrates. (Compare that to the WFPB diet's 8 to 12 percent from fat and 8 to 12 percent from protein.) This "Paleo" book and its imitators may soon become the most popular contenders in the low-carb genre, if they aren't already. So what's my take?

There are a number of low-carb gurus offering advice on how to eat, but, to my knowledge, Cordain is one of only two who have published in the peer-reviewed experimental research literature (the other being Eric Westman at Duke University), a practice that I strongly respect. So let's begin there, with Cordain's research.

Cordain bases his views on the highly conjectural dietary habits of the Paleo (Stone Age) people, as well as their contemporary counterparts, modern-day hunter-gatherers whose diets, he suggests, can be studied as surrogates for those eaten during Paleo times. However, he confesses in several places in his research papers[60] that estimates of dietary intakes in both of these groups are "subjective in nature." He also acknowledges that "scores" attempting to rate these presumed intakes from a very large compendium of 862 of the world's societies[61] "are not precise." Further, he notes that the true "hunter-gatherer way of life"—one not influenced by Western life—"is now probably extinct." Thus researchers "must rely on indirect procedures to reconstruct the traditional diet of pre-agricultural humans." This is an honest but rather apologetic view of this research.

Prior to 2000, anthropologists seemed to have reached a consensus, arising from a 1968 publication by Richard Lee,[62] that across fifty-eight different hunter-gatherer societies, only about 33 percent of the consumed foods were animal-based. In a research paper[63] in 2000, however, Cordain introduced a very different estimate. Unlike Lee, Cordain included fish in his definition of animal-based foods, and he added a larger number of hunter-gatherer societies for his review (229 as opposed to fifty-eight). Cordain then concluded that 66 to 75 percent of these "Paleo" diets represented animal-based foods—a proportion at least twice as high as Lee's earlier estimate.

By broadening the scope of his research in this way, Cordain substantially shifted the conversation. Now, instead of ancient dietary habits being regarded as primarily plant-based, they are considered to be animal-based. Cordain claims that his new estimate is supported by another, "more exacting" report[64] conducted on a smaller sample of hunter-gatherer societies, which concluded that 65 percent of these diets were animal-based— very close to Cordain's own estimate of 68 percent.

In his work, Cordain enthuses about humans being rather carnivorous, suggesting that "hominids may have experienced a number of genetic adaptations to animal-based diets early on in our genus's evolution analogous to those of obligate carnivores such as the feline."[65] He goes on to say that "even when plant food sources would have been available year round at lower [tropical] latitudes, animal foods would have been the preferred energy source of the majority of worldwide hunter-gatherers" and, further, that "the tissues of wild animals would have almost always represented the staple food for the world's contemporary hunter-gatherers." Like other low-carb proponents, Cordain regards the consumption of animal-based foods as an almost sacred part of the human tradition, with deep roots in our distant past.

Cordain's new interpretation of early human diets has been challenged, on several grounds, by the scientific literature. First, according to anthropologist Katherine Milton,[66] Cordain's assumption that contemporary hunter-gatherers are representative of historical hunter-gatherers could be a stretch. Most of the earlier hunter-gatherers had vanished or been pushed into marginal environments before present-day surveys on hunter-gatherers were collected (a view shared by Cordain[67]). Accordingly, it is questionable if these more recent hunter-gatherers are the "survivors [representing] the primitive condition of mankind."[68]

Second, Cordain's provocative idea that humans "may have experienced a number of genetic adaptations to animal-based diets" like carnivorous felines is really only a conjecture (note his use of "may have"). To my knowledge, there is no evidence that genetic adaptations favoring the consumption of animal-based foods could have occurred on the scale required to convert early humans into true carnivores.[69]

Third, humans cannot synthesize their own vitamin C, which is made only in plants. Other mammals that require vitamin C are all plant eaters; mammals whose diets are primarily carnivorous, in contrast, don't require it. Why would humans be any different?

Fourth, for most of their early history, humans did not have the speed or strength to catch and slaughter larger animals for food, making the possibility of diets high in animal protein rather low. (However, Cordain does make a reasonably plausible argument for the possibility that some prehistoric groups did regularly hunt animals, mostly dependent on the high energy return hunters would have received in exchange for the energy expended in hunting[70]).

Fifth, human anatomy compares well with that of our nearest living nonhuman primate relatives, like chimpanzees, who do and always have mostly relied on plants for dinner. We share a similar gut anatomy (simple acid stomach, a small intestine, a small cecum, and a markedly sacculated colon), and the diets of these near-relative nonhuman primates contain only 4 to 6 percent animal-based food, most of which consists of termites and ants.[71] (Cordain, in fact, presented a very similar estimate for the amount of meat in prehistoric humans' diets—3 to 5 percent—in a 2004 symposium in Denver, Colorado [a symposium that hosted a talk by me as well].)

These points taken together form a more than adequate argument against the reliability of Cordain's rather sweeping claims about the animal-food-oriented nature of prehistoric humans' diet. I cannot understand how the Paleo Diet enthusiasts are so certain of their views based on evidence that is so conjectural and uncertain—and so at odds with modern-day findings, obtained using research methodologies that are far more direct and robust. Using crude approximations of what ancient people may have eaten as primary evidence for what we should be eating today makes very little sense to me. Using evidence obtained from contemporary hunter-gatherer people as a surrogate raises the same uncertainty, especially when these contemporary groups' diets are likely to have been greatly altered from those of earlier times.

Also add to these concerns the highly questionable nature of animal-versus-plant-food dietary estimates taken from archaeological studies, given that plant foods leave little or no trace in fossilized remains. Further, what do we know about the lifespans of prehistoric people? Did they live long enough to suffer the diet-dependent degenerative diseases of aging? Evolutionary arguments that draw conclusions about health impacts beyond the ages of fertility, after one is no longer able to pass on one's genes, are not especially convincing, and if our ancestors did not live long enough to develop these diseases, then fossil remains cannot be used as evidence to draw conclusions about their long-term health.

I agree that humans must have consumed *some* amount of animal-based food during their evolutionary past. But I don't agree that we should use highly questionable evidence from ancient history to vigorously assert the correct amounts of protein and fat to be consumed in the present day, when we have access to far superior research methodologies and experimentation.

Like other low-carb advocates, Cordain fails to explain or even mention evidence that sharply contrasts with his hypothesis, especially evidence that supports the health value of the whole-food, plant-based diet. For example, it has long been established that when diet and disease correlations for different populations are compared (as in cross-sectional studies), diets rich in fat and animal protein (like the Paleo Diet) correlate strongly with higher rates of heart disease and cancers of the breast, colon, and prostate,[72] to name only a few. (Although I mention cross-sectional correlation studies, I am not inferring specific causality from these correlations; I am only saying that this long-established and indisputable relationship—the high ratio of animal to plant foods, expressed in various ways—categorically refutes the main tenet of the Paleo/low-carb advocates.) I know of no studies, for example, showing that a Paleo/low-carb diet is associated with lower rates of these and other related Western diseases. There is absolutely no wiggle room here.

Another profound effect that Cordain and other low-carb advocates ignore concerns the substantial health benefits that are quickly observed when people adopt a WFPB diet. When switching to the WFPB diet from the current American diet that is only marginally less high in fat and protein than the Paleo/low-carb diet, the health benefits are broad, surprisingly rapid, and relatively free of side effects. I know of no evidence yet produced showing that the Paleo/low-carb diet can do this, marking a truly striking difference between the Paleo/low-carb diet and the WFPB diet.

In general, when following the WFPB diet, serious illnesses like heart disease,[73] diabetes,[74] and certain cancers (including cancer of the liver[75] and pancreas[76] and melanoma[77]) and auto-immune diseases are not only prevented but, more important, can be intercepted in their forward progress and even reversed (as reviewed in *The China Study*). The evidence on treating these diseases has been published in peer-reviewed professional journals, and I am confident that, in the near future, these same benefits will be shown for a broad spectrum of additional disease conditions.

You can read much more in *The China Study* (as well as in popular books by physicians Dean Ornish,[78] Caldwell Esselstyn,[79] John McDougall,[80] Neal Barnard,[81] Joel Fuhrman,[82] Pamela Popper,[83] among many others), but the evidence is remarkably consistent: when eating the WFPB diet—a diet that is *exactly the opposite* of the Paleo Diet—the benefits begin quickly, slowing and often reversing a broad spectrum of diseases and illnesses. Has a Paleo/low-carb diet ever been shown to do this? No. Not ever. And while more formal, peer-reviewed research still needs to be done on the comprehensive effects of the WFPB diet, the experimental, observational, and clinical evidence provides a remarkable degree of consistency. This type of evidence profoundly trumps any theoretically mechanistic or "archeological" evidence the Paleo Diet has to offer.

# PREVIEW OF
# *WHOLE: RETHINKING THE*
# *SCIENCE OF NUTRITION*
### *T. Colin Campbell, PhD,*
### *with Howard Jacobson, PhD*

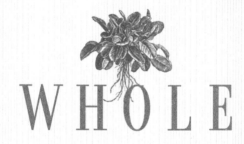

# WHOLE

### Rethinking the Science of Nutrition

Coauthor of international bestseller *The China Study*

## T. COLIN CAMPBELL, PhD

### with HOWARD JACOBSON, PhD

# INTRODUCTION

I n 1965, my academic career looked promising. After four years as a research associate at MIT, I was settling into my new office at Virginia Tech's Department of Biochemistry and Nutrition. Finally, I was a real professor! My research agenda couldn't have been more noble: end childhood malnutrition in poor countries by figuring out how to get more high-quality protein into their diets. My arena was the Philippines, thanks to a generous grant from the U.S. State Department's Agency for International Development.

The first challenge was to find a locally produced, inexpensive protein source. (Even though malnutrition is largely an issue of not getting enough calories overall, in the mid-1960s we thought that calories from protein were somehow special.) The second challenge was to develop a series of self-help centers around the country where we could show mothers how to raise their children out of malnutrition by using that protein source. My team and I chose peanuts, which are rich in protein and can grow under lots of different conditions.

At the same time, I was working on another project at the request of my department chair, Dean Charlie Engel. Charlie had secured U.S. Department of Agriculture funding to study aflatoxin, a cancer-causing chemical produced by a fungus, *Aspergillus flavus*, and my job was to learn all I could about how the fungus grew so we could prevent it from growing on various food sources. This was clearly an important project, as there was quite a bit of evidence that *Aspergillus flavus* caused liver cancer in lab rats (the mainstream assumption was, and still is to this day, that anything that causes cancer in rats or mice probably also causes cancer in humans).

I soon discovered that one of the main foods *Aspergillus flavus* contaminates is ... peanuts. In one of those cosmic coincidences that appears amazing only years later, I found myself studying peanuts in two completely different contexts simultaneously. And what I found when I looked deeply into these two seemingly unrelated issues (protein deficiency among the poor children of the Philippines and the conditions under which *Aspergillus flavus* grows) started to shake my world and caused me to question many of the bedrock assumptions on which I and most other nutritional scientists had built our careers.

Here's the main finding that turned my worldview—and ultimately, my world—upside down: the children in the Philippines who ate the highest-protein diets were the ones most likely to get liver cancer—even though the children with high-protein diets were significantly wealthier and had better access to all the things we typically associate with childhood health, like medical care and clean water.

I chose to follow this discovery everywhere it led me. As a result, the trajectory of my career veered in unexpected and unsettling directions, many of which are detailed in my first book, *The China Study*. I ultimately became aware of two things: First, nutrition is the master key to human health. Second, what most of us think of as proper nutrition *isn't*.

If you want to live free of cancer, heart disease, and diabetes for your entire life, that power is in your hands (and your knife and fork). But sadly, medical schools, hospitals, and government health agencies continue to treat nutrition as if it plays only a minor role in health. And no wonder: the standard Western diet, along with its trendy "low-fat" and "low-carb" cousins, is actually the cause, not the cure, of most of what ails us. In a nutshell, the "miracle cure" science has been chasing for the past half century turns out not to be a new wonder drug painstakingly formulated after decades of brilliant and relentless lab work or a cutting-edge surgical tool or technique using lasers and nanotechnology or some transformation of our DNA that will turn us all into immortal Apollos and Venuses. Instead, the secret of health has been in front of us all along, in the guise of a simple and perhaps boring word: nutrition. When it comes to our health, it turns out the trump card is the food we put in our mouths each day. In the process of learning all this, I also learned something else very important: why most people didn't know this already.

The medical and scientific research establishments, far from embracing these findings, have systematically dismissed and even suppressed them.

Few medical professionals are aware that our food choices can be far more effective shields against disease than the pills they prescribe.

Few health journalists report the unambiguous good news about radiant health and disease prevention through diet.

Few scientists are trained to look at the "big picture" and instead specialize in scrutinizing single drops of data instead of comprehending meaningful rivers of wisdom.

And paying the piper and calling the tune for all of them are the pharmaceutical and food industries, which are trying to convince us that salvation can be found in a pill or an enriched snack food made from plant fragments and artificial ingredients.

The truth. How it's been kept from you. And why. That's what this book is all about.

## Why Another Book?

If you've read *The China Study*, you've heard some of this before. You know the truth about nutrition, and you've heard a little bit about the resistance I and other scientists have faced in trying to bring this truth to light.

Since its publication in 2005, millions of people have read or read about *The China Study* and shared its insights with friends, neighbors, colleagues, and loved ones. Not a day goes by that I don't hear grateful testimonials to the healing power of whole, plant-based foods. Anecdotal as each of these stories may be, the overall weight of their combined evidence is substantial. And each of them is more than ample compensation for the troubles and obstacles placed in my way by powerful interests who make money from our collective ignorance.

Also, since 2005, many of my colleagues have conducted varied studies that show even more powerfully the effects of good eating on the various systems of the human body. At this point, any scientist, doctor, journalist, or policy maker who denies or minimizes the importance of a whole food, plant-based diet for individual and societal well-being simply isn't looking clearly at the facts. There's just too much good evidence to ignore anymore.

And yet, in some ways, very little has changed. Most people still don't know that the key to health and longevity is in their hands. Whether maliciously or, as is more often the case, due to ignorance, the mainstream of Western culture is hell-bent on ignoring, disbelieving, and, in some cases, actively twisting the truth about what we should be eating—so much so that it can be hard for us to believe that we've been lied to all these years. It's often easier to simply accept what we've been told, rather than consider the possibility of a conspiracy of control, silence, and misinformation. And the only way to combat this perception is to show you how and why it happened.

That's why this new book felt necessary. *The China Study* focused on the evidence that tells us the whole food, plant-based diet is the healthiest human diet. *Whole* focuses on why it's been so hard to bring that evidence to light—and on what still needs to happen for real change to take place.

## *WHOLE*: THE SUM OF ITS PARTS

This book is split into four parts.

The first, Part I, provides a little more information about my and others' research on the whole food, plant-based diet, my reflections on some of the most prominent criticisms this research has received since the publication of *The China Study*, and more of my own background and journey, as context for understanding where the philosophies in this book have come from.

Part II looks at the reason it's so hard for so many to not just accept, but even notice, the health implications of this research: the mental prison, or paradigm, in which Western science and medicine operate, which makes it impossible to see the obvious facts that lie outside it. For many reasons, we now operate under a paradigm that looks for truth only in the smallest details, while entirely ignoring the big picture. The popular expression "can't see the forest for the trees" makes the point well, except that there's much more at stake here than just trees and forests. Modern science is so detail obsessed that we can't see the forest for the vascular cambium and secondary phloem and so on. There's nothing wrong with looking at details (I spent most of my research career doing just that); the trouble occurs when we start denying that there *is* a big picture and stubbornly insist that the narrow reality we see, heavily laden with our own biases and experiences, is all there is.

The fancy word for this obsession with minutiae is *reductionism*. And reductionism comes with its own seductive logic, so that people laboring under its spell can't even see that there's another way to look at the world. To reductionists, all other worldviews are unscientific, superstitious, sloppy, and not worthy of attention. All evidence gathered by nonreductionist means—presuming that research can get funding in the first place—is ignored or suppressed.

Part III looks at the other side of this equation: the economic forces that reinforce and exploit this paradigm for their own self-interest as they chase financial success. These forces completely manipulate the public conversation about health and nutrition to suit their bottom line. We'll look at the many ways money affects thousands of small decisions that add up to a big impact on what you, the public, hear (and don't hear) and thus believe about health and nutrition.

Last, in Part IV, we look at the totality of what's at stake here and what's needed if we want things to change.

# THE TRUTH BELONGS TO ALL OF US

I wanted to tell this story because I owe it to you, the public. If you are a U.S. taxpayer, you paid for my career in research, teaching, and policy making. I have known too many people, including friends and family, who suffered ill health unnecessarily, just because they did not know what I have come to know—and they also were taxpayers. You have a right to know what your money bought and a right to benefit from its findings.

My own disclaimer: I have no financial interest in your believing me. I don't sell health products, health seminars, or health coaching. I'm seventy-nine years old, I've had a long and rewarding career, and I'm not writing this book to make a buck. When you start talking about what you've learned from this book with your friends and you encounter passionate disdain for me and my motives (and you will!), just consider the original source of the claims they're citing. Ask yourself: What's their financial interest? What do they have to gain from suppressing the information I share here?

Telling this story has been a challenge. I know well that a diet consisting only of plants sounds like a wacky idea to many folks. But that's starting to change. This idea becomes bigger and bigger with the passing of time. The current system is unsustainable. The only question is, will we free ourselves before it takes us down with it? Or will we continue to pollute our bodies, our minds, and our planet with the slag of that system until it collapses under its own economic weight and biological logic?

In previous generations, how we ate appeared to be a personal and private matter. Our food choices didn't seem to contribute much, one way or the other, to the well-being or suffering of other people, let alone animals, plant life, and the carrying capacity of the entire planet. But even if that were ever true, it no longer is. What we eat, individually and collectively, has repercussions far beyond our waistlines and blood pressure readings. No less than our future as a species hangs in the balance.

The choice is ours. My hope is that this book will encourage you to choose wisely—for your health, for the next generations, and for the entire planet.

# ACKNOWLEDGMENTS

I am indebted to Leah Wilson for her expert editing and to Howard Jacobson, my coauthor, both of whom made this book much more readable.

# ABOUT THE AUTHORS

For more than fifty years, **T. Colin Campbell, PhD**, has been at the forefront of nutrition research, authoring more than 300 professional research papers. His legacy, *The China Study*, coauthored with his son, Thomas Campbell, II, MD, has been a continuous international bestseller since its publication in 2005. He holds the position of Jacob Gould Schurman Professor Emeritus of Nutritional Biochemistry at Cornell University, has coauthored several expert food and health policy reports, and has lectured extensively worldwide on resolving the health care crisis through the little-known but remarkable effects of nutrition. He has founded a unique and highly successful set of online courses on plant-based nutrition as a partnership between the T. Colin Campbell Foundation (tcolincampbell.org) and Cornell University's online subsidiary, eCornell.

**Howard Jacobson, PhD**, is an online marketing consultant, health educator, and ecological gardener from Durham, North Carolina. He earned a Masters of Public Health and a Doctor of Health Studies from Temple University and a BA in history from Princeton. Howard runs an online marketing agency and is the author of *Google AdWords for Dummies*. He speaks, coaches, and consults on individual health and planetary sustainability and can be reached at howard@permanator.com.

# ENDNOTES

1. Harvard School of Public Health "Adult Obesity," http://www.hsph .harvard.edu/obesity-prevention-source/obesity-trends/obesity-rates-worldwide/

2. CDC: "Adult Obesity Facts," last modifed August 16, 2013, http://www .cdc.gov/obesity/data/adult.html.

3. To get the full effect of this data (an animated year-by-year march toward obesity), visit http://www.cdc.gov/obesity/data/adult.html and play the slideshow toward the bottom of the page.

4. Foster G.D., Wyatt H.R., Hill J.O., McGuckin B.G., Brill C., Mohammed B.S., Szapary P.O., Rader D.J., Edman J.S., and Klein S.: "A randomized trial of a low-carbohydrate diet for obesity," *New Engl J Med* 2003, 348: 2082–2090; Stern L., Iqbal N., Seshadri P., Chicano K.L., Daily D.A., McGrory J., Williams M., Gracely E.J., Samaha F.F.: "The effects of low-carbohydrate versus conventional weight loss diets in severely obese adults: one-year follow-up of a randomized trial," *Ann Internal Med* 2004, 140: 778–785; Carroll K.K., Braden L.M., Bell J.A., Kalamegham R.: "Fat and cancer," *Cancer* 1986, 58: 1818–1825.

5. At the time of his death, Atkins had wrestled with obesity and cardiac problems for many years, suffering cardiac arrest one year before his passing. When he died, Atkins was 258 pounds and 6 feet tall, which classifies him as obese. If Atkins was not following his own diet, then I must ask why not.

6. Yancy Jr. W.S., Olsen M.K., Guyton J.R., Bakst R.P., and Westman E.C.: "A low-carbohydrate, ketogenic diet versus a low-fat diet to treat obesity and hyperlipidemia," *Ann Internal Med* 2004, 140: 769–777.

7. Westman E.C., Yancy W.S., Edman J.S., Tomlin K.F., and Perkins, C.E.: "Effect of 6-month adherence to a very low carbohydrate diet program," *Am. J Med* 2002, 113: 30–36.

8. Kritchevsky D.: "Caloric restriction and cancer," *J Nutr Sci Vitaminol* 2001, 47: 13–19.

9. Hegsted D.M., in *Present Knowledge of Nutrition* (D.M. Hegsted et al., eds) 1 (Nutrition Foundation, 4th ed., 1976).

10. Campbell T.C. and Chen J.: "Characteristics in rural China: lessons learned and unlearned," *Nutr Today* 1999, 34: 116–123.

11. Rippe J.M. and Angelopoulos T.J.: "Sucrose, high-fructose corn syrup, and fructose, their metabolism and potential health effects: What do we really know?" *Adv Nutr* 2013, 4: 236–245.

12. Bray G.A.: "Energy and fructose from beverages sweetened with sugar or high-fructose corn syrup pose a health risk for some people," *Adv Nutr* 2013, 4: 220–225.

13. Satija A. and Hu F.B.: "Cardiovascular benefits of dietary fiber," *Curr Atheroscler Rep* 2012, 14: 505–514.

14. Kritchevsky D.: "Calories and chemically induced tumors in rodents," *Comprehensive Therapy* 1985, 11: 35–39.

15. Horio F., Youngman L.D., Bell R.C., and Campbell T. C.: "Thermogenesis, low-protein diets, and decreased development of AFB1-induced preneoplastic foci in rat liver," *Nutr. Cancer* 1991, 16: 31–41.

16. Krieger E.: "Increased voluntary exercise by Fisher 344 rats fed low-protein diets," Undergraduate Thesis, *Cornell University* (1988).

17. Miller D.S. and Payne P.R.: "Weight maintenance and food intake," *J Nutr* 1962, 78: 255–262.

18. Chen J., Campbell T.C., Li J., and Peto R.: "Diet, Lifestyle and Mortality in China: A Study of the Characteristics of 65 Chinese Counties" (Oxford University Press; Cornell University Press; People's Medical Publishing House: 1990).

19. Campbell T.C. and Chen J.: "Energy balance: Interpretation of data from rural China," *Toxicol Sci* 1999, 52 (suppl): 87–94.

20. Rothwell N.J. and Stock M.J.: "Regulation of energy balance," *Ann Rev Nutr* 1981, 1: 235–256; Rothwell N.J. and Stock M.J.: "Influence of carbohydrate and fat intake on diet-induced thermogenesis and brown fat activity in rats fed low protein diets," *J Nutr* 1987, 117: 1721–1726; Rothwell N.J., Stock M.J., and Tyzbir R.S.: "Mechanisms of thermogenesis induced by low-protein diets," *Metabolism* 1983, 32: 257–261.

21. Taubes uses two reference lists: the first is a list of annotations, which are only linked to page numbers and a few key words or phrases that must be found on the page, and the second is merely an alphabetized bibliography. In effect, there is no direct one-to-one linkage between text citation and bibliography, so it is not obvious when a comment in the text is even being referenced.

22. Not to be confused with brown adipose tissue, mentioned earlier.

23. Keys A.: "Coronary heart disease in seven countries," *Circulation Suppl* 1970, 41: I1–I211.

24. Keys A.: *Seven Countries: A Multivariate Analysis of Death and Coronary Heart Disease* (Cambridge, Harvard University Press: 1980).

25. CDC: "Morbidity and Morality Weekly Report," 48(30);651, last modified May 2, 2001, http://www.cdc.gov/mmwr/preview/mmwrhtml/mm4830a1box.htm.

26. Keys A.: "The diet/heart controversy," *Lancet* 1979: 844–845.

27. Keys A.: "Coronary heart disease—the global picture," *Atherosclerosis* 1975, 22: 149–192.

28. NAS: "Diet, Nutrition and Cancer Report," 1982.

29. Kennedy E.T., Bowman S.A., and Powell R.: "Dietary fat intake in the US population," *Journal Am Coll Nutr* 1999, 18: 207–212.

30. Ibid.

31. Select Committee on Nutrition and Human Needs (U.S. Senate): *Dietary goals for the United States*, 2nd edition, 83 (U.S. Government Printing Office, Washington, D.C.: 1977).

32. Ibid.

33. As an aside, that was when I learned that DeVita's estimate of funding for diet and cancer research at NCI, which funded our research, was limited to an appalling 2–3% of the total budget.

34. Committee on Diet Nutrition and Cancer: "Diet, Nutrition and Cancer" (Washington, D.C., National Academy Press: 1982).

35. Council for Agricultural Science and Technology: "Diet, nutrition and cancer: A critique," special publication no. 13 80 (Iowa, Council for Agricultural Science and Technology: 1982).

36. Committee on Diet Nutrition and Cancer: "Diet, Nutrition and Cancer" (Washington, D.C., National Academy Press: 1982).

37. United States Department of Health and Human Services: "The Surgeon General's Report on Nutrition and Health" (Dallas, Superintendent of Documents, U.S. Government Printing Office: 1988).

38. National Research Council & Committee on Diet and Health: "Diet and health: Implications for reducing chronic disease risk" (Washington, D.C., National Academy Press: 1989).

39. Expert Panel: "Food, nutrition and the prevention of cancer: A global perspective" (Washington, D.C., American Institute for Cancer Research/World Cancer Research Fund: 1997).

40. Kritchevsky D., Tepper S.A., Davidson L.M., and Fisher E.A.: "Experimental atherosclerosis in rabbits fed cholesterol-free diets: 13-Interaction of proteins and fat," *Atherosclerosis* 1989, 75: 123–127.

41. Kritchevsky D.: "Vegetable protein and atherosclerosis," *J Am Oil Chem Soc* 1979, 56: 135; Carroll K.K. and Hamilton R.M.G.: "Effects of dietary protein and carbohydrate on plasma cholesterol levels in relation to atherosclerosis," *J Food Sci* 1975, 40: 18; Terpstra A.H., Harkes L., and Van Der Veen F.H.: "The effect of different proportions of casein in semipurified diets on the concentration of serum cholesterol and the lipoprotein compostion in rabbits," *Lipids* 1981, 16: 114–119; Kritchevsky D., Tepper S.A., Czarnecki S.K., and Klurfeld D.M.: "Experimental atherosclerosis in rabbits fed cholesterol-free diets," *Atherosclerosis* 1981, 39: 169.

42. Meeker D.R. and Kesten H.D.: "Experimental atherosclerosis and high protein diets," *Proc Soc Exp Biol Med* 1940, 45: 543–545; Meeker D.R. and Kesten H.D.: "Effect of high protein diets on experimental atherosclerosis of rabbits," *Arch Pathology* 1941, 31: 147–162.

43. Hodges R.E., Krehl W.A., Stone D.B., and Lopez A.: "Dietary carbohydrates and low-cholesterol diets: Effects on serum lipids of man," *Am J Clin Nutr* 1967, 20: 198–208; Sirtori C.R., Agradi E., Conti F., Mantero O., and Gatti E.: "Soybean-protein diet in the treatment of type II hyperlipoproteinemia," *Lancet* 1977, 1(8006): 275–277; Forsythe W.A., Green M.S., and Amderson J.J.B.: "Dietary protein effects on cholesterol and lipoprotein concentrations: a review," *J Am Coll Nutr* 1986, 5: 533–549.

44. Youngman L.D.: "The growth and development of aflatoxin B1-induced preneoplastic lesions, tumors, metastasis, and spontaneous tumors as

they are influenced by dietary protein level, type, and intervention" (Cornell University, PhD thesis: 1990).

45. Sanchez A. and Hubbard R.W.: "Plasma amino acids and the insulin/ glucagon ratio as an explanation for the dietary protein modulation of atherosclerosis," *Med Hypoth* 1991, 36: 27–32.

46. Walker G.R., Morse E.H., and Overlay V.A.: "The effect of animal protein and vegetable protein diets having the same fat content on the serum lipid levels of young women," *J Nutr* 1960, 72: 317–321.

47. Sirtori C.R., Agradi E., Conti F., Mantero O., and Gatti, E.: "Soybean-protein diet in the treatment of type II hyperlipoproteinemia," *Lancet* 1977, 1 (8006): 275–277.

48. Carroll K.K.: "Hypercholesterolemia and atherosclerosis: effects of dietary protein," *Fed Proc* 1982, 41: 2792–2796; Sirtori C.R. et al.: "Clinical experience with soybean-protein diet in the treatment of hypercholesterolemia," *Am J Clin Nutr* 1979, 31: 1645–1658; Descovich G.C. et al., in "Lipoproteins and coronary atherosclerosis," Symposium Giovanni Lorenzini Foundation (Noseda G., Fragiacomo C., Fumagali R., and Paoletti R., eds), 279 (Amsterdam, Elsevier Biomedical Press: 1982); Goldberg A.P. et al.: "Soybean protein independently lowers plasma cholesterol levels in primary hypercholesterolemia," *Atherosclerosis* 1982, 43: 355–368.

49. Hession M., Rolland C., Kulkarni U., Wise A., and Broom J.: "Systematic review of raondomized controlled trials of low-carbohydrate vs. low-fat/low-calorie diets in the management of obesity and its comorbidities," *Obesity Rev* 2009, 10: 36–50.

50. Gardner C.D. et al.: "Comparison of the Atkins, Zone, Ornish, and LEARN diets for change in weight and related risk factors among overweight premenopausal women: The A to Z weight loss study: A randomized trial," *JAMA* 2007, 297: 969–977.

51. Brownell K.D.: *The LEARN Manual for Weight Management* (Euless, Texas, American Health Publishing Company: 2000).

52. Sears B.: *The Zone* (New York: Harpers Collins Publishers: 1995).

53. Estruch R., Ros E., Salas-Salvado J., Covas M-I., Corella D., Aros F., Gome-Garcia E., Ruiz-Getoerrez V., Fiol M., Lapetra J., et al.: "Primary prevention of cardiovascular disease with a Mediterranean diet," NEJM 2013, 368.

54. "Supplementary Appendix" to Estruch R. et al.: "Primary Prevention of cardiovascular disease." http://www.nejm.org/doi/suppl/10.1056/NEJMoa1200303/suppl_file/nejmoa1200303_appendix.pdf.

55. Bravata D.M., Sanders L., Huang J., Krumholz H.M., Olkin I., and Gardner C.D.: "Efficacy and safety of low-carbohydrate diets: A systematic review," *JAMA* 2003, 289: 1837–1850.

56. Nordmann A.J., Nordmann A., Briel M., Keller U., Yancy W.S., Brehm B.J., and Bucher H.C.: "Effects of low-carbohydrate vs low-fat diets on weight loss and cardiovascular risk factors," *Arch Intern Med* 2006, 166: 285–293.

57. Hession M., Rolland C., Kulkarni U., Wise A., and Broom J.: "Systematic review of randomized controlled trials of low-carbohydrate vs. low-fat/low-calorie diets in the management of obesity and its comorbidities," *Obesity Rev* 2009, 10: 36–50.

58. Gardner C.D. et al., "Comparison of the Atkins, Zone, Ornish, and LEARN diets."

59. Noto H., Goto A., Tsujimoto T., and Noda M.: "Low-carbohydrate diets and all-cause mortality: a systematic review and meta-analysis of observational studies," *PLoS ONE* 2013, 8: 1–10.

60. Cordain L., Brand Miller J., Eaton S.B., Mann N., Holt S.H.A., and Speth J.D.: "Plant-animal subsistence ratios and macronutrient energy estimations in worldwide hunter-gatherer diets," *Am J Clin Nutr* 2000, 71: 682–692; Cordain L., Eaton S.B., Miller J.B., Mann N., and Hill K.: "The paradoxical nature of hunter-gatherer diets: Meat-based, yet non-atherogenic," *European J Clin Nutr* 2002, 56: S42–S52.

61. Murdock G.P.: "Ethnographic atlas: A summary," *Ethnology* 1967, 6: 109–236.

62. Lee R.B.: *What Humans Do for a Living, Or How to Make Out on Scarce Resources* (Chicago, IL, Aldine Publishing House: 1968).

63. Cordain L., Brand Miller J., Eaton S.B., Mann N., Holt S.H.A., and Speth J.D.: "Plant-animal subsistence ratios and macronutrient energy estimations in worldwide hunter-gatherer diets," *Am J Clin Nutr* 2000, 71: 682–692.

64. Kaplan H., Hill K., Lancaster J., and Hurtado A.M.: "A theory of human life history evolution: Diet, intelligence, and longevity," *Evol Anthropol* 2000, 9: 156–185.

65. Cordain L., Eaton S.B., Miller J.B., Mann N., and Hill K.: "The paradoxical nature of hunter-gatherer diets: Meat-based, yet non-atherogenic," *European J Clin Nutr* 2002, 56: S42–S52.

66. Milton K.: "Hunter-gatherer diets—A different perspective," *Am J Clin Nutr* 2000, 71: 665–667.

67. Cordain L., Brand Miller J., Eaton S.B., Mann N., Holt S.H.A., and Speth J.D.: "Plant-animal subsistence ratios and macronutrient energy estimations in worldwide hunter-gatherer diets," *Am J Clin Nutr* 2000, 71: 682–692.

68. Isaac G.L.I. and Crader D.C.: "To what extent were early hominids carnivorous? An archeological perspective," In *Omnivorous Primates: Gathering and Hunting in Human Evolution* edited by Harding R.S.O. and Teleki G. (New York: Columbia University Press: 1981), 37–103.

69. Draper H.H.: "The aboriginal Eskimo diet in modern perspective," *Am Anthropol* 1977, 79: 309–316; Ho K.J., Mikkelson B., Lewis L.A., Feldman S.A., and Taylor C.B.: "Alaskan Arctic Eskimos: Responses to a customary high-fat diet," *Am J Clin Nutr* 1972, 25: 737–745.

70. Cordain L., Brand Miller J., Eaton S.B., Mann N., Holt S.H.A., and Speth J.D.: "Plant-animal subsistence ratios and macronutrient energy estimations in worldwide hunter-gatherer diets," *Am J Clin Nutr* 2000, 71: 682–692.

71. Milton K.: "Nutritional characteristics of wild primate foods: Do the diets of our closest living relatives have lessons for us?" *Nutrition* 1999, 15: 488–498.

72. Carroll K.K.: "Experimental evidence of dietary factors and hormone-dependent cancers," *Cancer Res* 1975, 35: 3374–3383; World Cancer Research Fund/American Institute for Cancer Research: *Food, Nutrition, Physical Activity, and Prevention of Cancer: A Global Perspective* (Washington, D.C., American Institute for Cancer Research: 2007).

73. Esselstyn C.B.: "Updating a 12-year experience with arrest and reversal therapy for coronary heart disease (an overdue requiem for palliative cardiology)," *Am J Cardiology* 1999, 84: 339–341; Morrison L.M.: "Diet in coronary atherosclerosis," *JAMA* 1960, 173: 884–888; Ornish D., Brown S.E., Scherwitz L.W., Billings J.H., Armstrong W.T., Ports T.A., McLanahan S.M., Kirkeeide R.L., Brand R.J., and Gould K.L.:

"Can lifestyle changes reverse coronary heart disease?" *Lancet* 1990, 336: 129–133.

74. Barnard R.J., Lattimore L., Holly R.G., Cherny S., and Pritikin N.: "Response of non-insulin-dependent diabetic patients to an intensive program of diet and exercise," *Diabetes Care* 1982, 5: 370–374.

75. Youngman L.D. and Campbell T.C.: "Inhibition of aflatoxin B1-induced gamma-glutamyl transpeptidase positive (GGT+) hepatic preneoplastic foci and tumors by low protein diets: evidence that altered GGT+ foci indicate neoplastic potential," *Carcinogenesis* 1992, 13: 1607–1613.

76. O'Connor T.P., Roebuck B.D., and Campbell T.C.: "Dietary intervention during the post-dosing phase of L-azaserine-induced preneoplastic lesions," *J Natl Cancer Inst* 1985, 75: 955–957.

77. Hildenbrand G.L.G., Hildenbrand L.C., Bradford K. and Cavin S.W.: "Five-year survival rates of melanoma patients treated by diet therapy after the manner of Gerson: a retrospective review," *Alternative Therapies in Health and Medicine* 1995, 1: 29–37.

78. Ornish D.: *Dr. Dean Ornish's Program for Reversing Heart Disease* (New York, Random House: 1990).

79. Esselstyn C.J.: *Prevent and Reverse Heart Disease* (New York, Avery Publishing, Penguin Group: 2007).

80. McDougall J.: *The Starch Solution* (New York, Rodale Press: 2012).

81. Barnard N.: *21-Day Weight Loss Kickstart: Boost Metabolism, Lower Cholesterol, and Dramatically Improve Your Health* (New York, Grand Central Lifestyle: 2011).

82. Fuhrman J.: *Eat to Live: The Revolutionary Formula for Fast and Sustained Weight Loss* (Boston, Little, Brown and Company: 2003).

83. Popper P., Merzer G., and Sroufe D.: *Food Over Medicine: The Conversation That Could Save Your Life* (Dallas, TX, BenBella Books: 2013).

# INDEX

"I have often been asked—a few hundred times, I think—what do my family and I eat? . . . Now I am happy to say that there is a cookbook that comes about as close to the real deal for our family as I can imagine it. This is it."
—T. COLIN CAMPBELL, PhD, coauthor of *The China Study*

LeAnne Campbell, daughter of *The China Study*'s T. Colin Campbell, delivers easily prepared and delicious recipes that support optimal nutrition in . . .

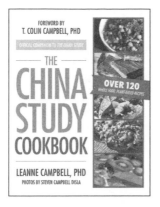

# The China Study Cookbook

## Over 120 Whole Food, Plant-Based Recipes

By LEANNE CAMPBELL, PhD

*The China Study Cookbook* takes the vital scientific findings from *The China Study* and puts the science into action. Written by LeAnne Campbell, PhD, daughter of *The China Study* coauthor T. Colin Campbell, PhD, and mother of two hungry teenagers, *The China Study Cookbook* features delicious, easily prepared plant-based recipes. From her Fabulous Sweet Potato Enchiladas to No-Bake Peanut Butter Bars, all of LeAnne's recipes have no added fat and minimal sugar and salt to promote optimal health. Filled with helpful tips on substitutions, keeping foods nutrient-rich, and transitioning to a plant-based diet, *The China Study Cookbook* shows how to transform individual health and the health of the entire family.

LEANNE CAMPBELL, PhD, has been preparing meals based on a whole food, plant-based diet for almost 20 years. Campbell has raised two sons—Steven and Nelson, now 18 and 17—on this diet. As a working mother, she has found ways to prepare quick and easy meals without using animal products or adding fat.

Visit THECHINASTUDY.COM and THECHINASTUDYCOOKBOOK.COM to learn more!

From the author of the groundbreaking
bestseller, *The China Study*, comes the much-anticipated ...

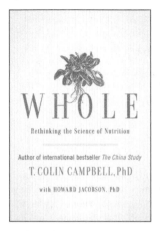

# WHOLE
## Rethinking the Science of Nutrition

By T. COLIN CAMPBELL, PhD
and HOWARD JACOBSON, PhD

*Whole* picks up where *The China Study* left off. *The China Study* revealed what we should eat and provided the powerful empirical support for this answer. *Whole* answers *why* a whole food, plant-based diet provides optimal nutrition. *Whole* demonstrates how far the scientific reductionism of the nutrition orthodoxy has gotten off track and reveals the elegant holistic workings of nutrition, from the cellular level to the operation of the entire organism. *Whole* is a marvelous journey through cutting-edge thinking on nutrition, led by one of the masters of the science.

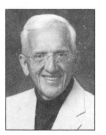

For more than 40 years, T. COLIN CAMPBELL, PhD, has been at the forefront of nutrition research. His legacy, the China Study, is the most comprehensive study of health and nutrition ever conducted. Dr. Campbell is the coauthor of the bestselling book *The China Study* and the Jacob Gould Schurman Professor Emeritus of Nutritional Biochemistry at Cornell University. He has received more than 70 grant-years of peer-reviewed research funding and authored more than 300 research papers. *The China Study* was the culmination of a 20-year partnership of Cornell University, Oxford University, and the Chinese Academy of Preventive Medicine.

Visit **THECHINASTUDY.COM** to learn more!